Medicinal Herbs in the Bible

Medicinal Herbs
in the
Bible

Dr. M. de Waal

Samuel Weiser, Inc.
York Beach, Maine

First published in Dutch in 1980 by
Uitgeverij Schors
Amsterdam, Holland
under the title *Geneeskruiden in de Bijbel*
Copyright © 1980 W. N. Schors

First published in the United States in 1984 by
Samuel Weiser, Inc.
Box 612
York Beach, ME 03910

Reprinted, 1988

English translation copyright © Samuel Weiser, Inc., 1984

All rights reserved. No part of this publication may be reproduced
or transmitted in any form or by any means, electronic or mechanical,
including photocopy, without permission in writing from the publisher.
Reviewers may quote brief passages.

ISBN 0-87728-527-6
Library of Congress Catalog Card Number: 84-52093

English translation by Jane Meijlink-Green

Printed in the United States of America

Contents

A Note to the Reader.................................ix
Introduction 1
Roots... 15
Woods and Barks..................................... 29
Herbs.. 41
Fruits and Seeds 57
Fibers and Amorphous Raw Materials 79
Animal Products...................................... 99
Bibliography 105
Index... 107

List of Illustrations

Gathering Herbs 2
Mandrake Root 16
Acacia Tree. 30
Indian Hemp 42
Lemon Tree. 58
Aloe 80
Honey. 100

A Note to the Reader

Dr. Marinus de Waal was born in 1876, and was a Professor of Comparative Religion at the University of Nÿmegen in Holland. The extensive research that resulted in *Medicinal Herbs in the Bible* was based upon the Dutch Leiden translation of the Bible, and also upon several now rare texts on botany, herbology and pharmacology. For the reader interested in continuing research, we have provided these original reference works at the back of the book. Many of them are now out of print, but may be found in library archives.

In preparing this translation for the American reader, the following translations of the Bible were used:

For all quotes from the Old Testament, the reader is referred to *The Holy Scriptures According to the Masoretic Text* (The Jewish Publication Society of America).

For quotes from the New Testament and from the Apocrypha, the reader is referred to *The New English Bible with the Apocrypha* (Oxford University Press).

The Publisher

INTRODUCTION

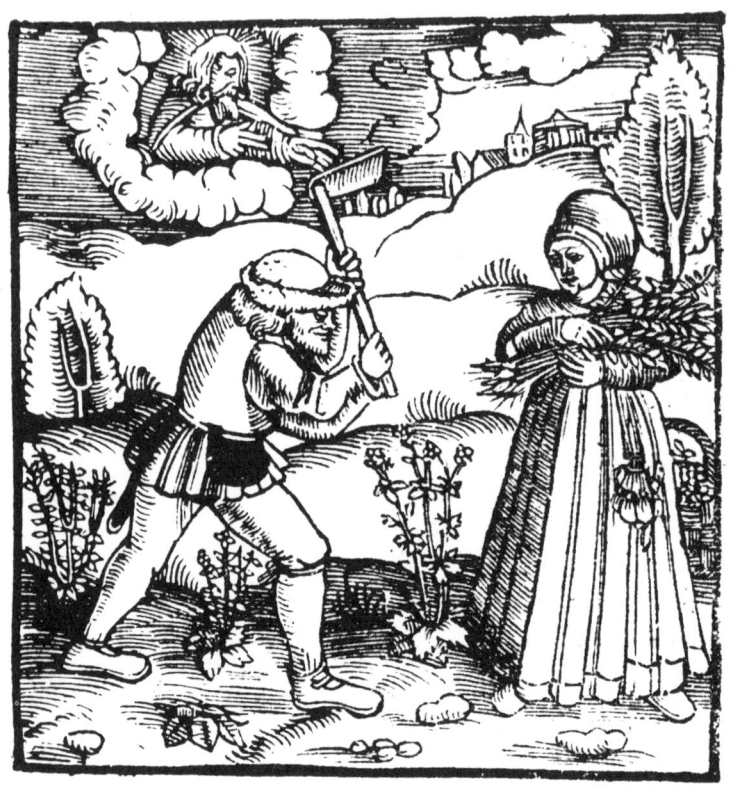

The Lord hath created medicines out of the earth; and he that is wise will not abhor them.

(Ecclesiasticus 38:4)
From Adam Lonicer, "Kreuterbuch" 1564.

Biblical Medicine

It should come as no surprise that some of the "simples" (herbs) used today played an important role as food, seasoning and medicine in the daily life of the people who lived in the mountainous country of ancient Palestine. Many of the remedies we use come to us from these primitive peoples who, seeking medicine for their own illnesses, have provided us with insight into the beneficial properties of many parts of plants or animals.

However, use of medicinal herbs was not an outgrowth of the Hebrew's knowledge of medicine, for in fact such knowledge did not then exist. Use of herbs for medicinal purposes grew out of extremely high standards for hygiene, as laid down by the law of Moses. Medical knowledge was of little significance in comparison with the social hygiene discussed in the Pentateuch (the first five books of the Old Testament) ascribed to Moses. We must keep in mind that we cannot always learn from ancient medical practices, since a considerable gulf divides ancient and modern conceptions and descriptions of illnesses—the result is that the significance of many texts written in classical antiquity are no longer comprehensible. The situation is even worse when one considers the obscure methods of curing illnesses. But the law of Moses is a unique phenomenon which loses nothing of its value in light of modern science, and the health practices prescribed therein are still applicable today. Consider, for example, the continuing value of the laws governing diet and food preparation, prophylaxis, the fight against venereal disease, and the institution of the Sabbath.[1]

The fact that medical *knowledge* in the time of the prophets (approximately 900-500 B.C.) was not far advanced is due to the fact that medical *miracles* were accepted, as can be seen in the miraculous cures of Elijah, Elisha and Isaiah. Medicine may have formed part of the curriculum in the prophets' schools, but the prophets were never considered to be healers. Because of the religious nature of the law of Moses, the Levites (the priests) became health officials and probably spread their knowledge by oral tradition. There must have been professional physicians in their time, however, as indicated by biblical references.

> Is there no balm in Gilead?
> Is there no physician there?
> (Jeremiah 8:22)

Physicians

Physician probably comes from the Hebrew *rôphê,* derived from a stem which means "alleviate" or "calm." Another explanation for its derivation is that it comes from the Arabic *raphâ,* "to sew." A physician, therefore, would be a "sewer" of wounds. The word *rôphê* first appears in the Bible when Jacob, the father of Joseph, is embalmed by his servants: "And Joseph commanded his servants the physicians to embalm his father." (Genesis 50:2). It is evident from the proverbs of Sirach that by 200 B.C. physicians were already held in respect:

> Honour the doctor for his services,
> for the Lord created him.

---

[1] The institution of the Sabbath had important ramifications in terms of health: on the seventh day one fasted, and took time off from all work to rest. In our present day society, this day of rest is one of the most important ways of reducing stress, which is a major cause of disease.

> His skill comes from the Most High,
> and he is rewarded by kings.
> (Ecclesiasticus 38:1, 2)

The doctrine brought forth by the followers of Sirach, that the physician is an instrument in the hands of the Lord to fulfill divine will, explains the apparent contradiction between predestination and intervention on the part of the physician.

Medicine was fairly advanced in Egypt; the Israelites, who spent a long period there, brought with them this knowledge, and physicians were held in respect for some time. However, in the centuries before the birth of Christ, there were, unquestionably, fluctuations in the esteem in which medical practice was held. It is said that Asa, King of Judah (923-883 B.C.), sought help not from the Lord but from the physicians:

> And in the thirty and ninth year of his reign Asa was diseased in his feet; his disease was exceeding great; yet in his disease he sought not to the Lord, but to the physicians.
> (II Chronicles 16:12)

But their help was of no avail since he had not sought the support of God. This is also apparent in a passage from Exodus, where the Lord is described as a healer:

> ... 'If thou wilt diligently hearken to the voice of the Lord thy God, and wilt do that which is right in His eyes, and wilt give ear to His commandments, and keep all His statutes, I will put none of the diseases upon thee, which I have put upon the Egyptians; for I am the Lord that healeth thee.'
> (Exodus 15:26)

In the law of Moses further on in Exodus, it is not entirely clear if it specifically means that the cost of a physician must be paid by the one who causes injury to another:

> And if men contend, and one smite the other with a stone, or with his fist, and he die not, but keep his

> bed; if he rise again, and walk abroad upon his staff, then shall he that smote him be quit; only he shall pay for the loss of his time, and shall cause him to be thoroughly healed.
>
> (Exodus 21:18, 19)

This could mean payment for a nurse, without the individual specifically being a physician.

In the New Testament, Jesus and his disciples are portrayed as physicians who help the sick by means of miracles. St. Mark refers to professional physicians who had not succeeded in curing a woman who was healed by touching the garments of Jesus:

> Among them was a woman who had suffered from haemorrhages for twelve years; and in spite of long treatment by many doctors, on which she had spent all she had, there had been no improvement; on the contrary, she had grown worse.
>
> (Mark 5:25, 26)

St. Luke himself must likewise have been a physician: "Greetings to you from our dear friend Luke, the doctor, and from Demas." (Colossians 4:14). Recognition of the necessity for medical help is apparent from the metaphors used by Jesus when asked why he and his disciples sat at table with publicans and sinners: "It is not the healthy that need a doctor, but the sick . . ." (Luke 5:31)

Later on in Hebrew tradition, a doctor was appointed to the temple to care for the ceremonial officials who suffered many complaints of the lower part of the body due to the innumerable washings and walking barefoot.

The doctor in biblical times was both a surgeon and his own apothecary. He had nothing to do with confinements, which were handled exclusively by midwives.

Illness

There are direct references to many specific illnesses in the Bible although the same name is frequently given to many complaints. These would include such illnesses as skin diseases, mental disorders, etc., each of which now have their own name. Fever, scabies, plague, leprosy, tuberculosis, blindness, paralysis, caries, dysentery and worm diseases are all discussed in different parts of the Holy Scriptures. Due to a fear of being made unclean by touching dead bodies, anatomical studies were not made by the Israelites, and as a consequence fine distinctions were not made within each type of ailment.

Methods of Healing and Medicine

Methods of healing are only given for a few illnesses, and references to these methods are infrequent in the Bible. Although a number of water baths and some plant and animal products are mentioned, reference is generally made to medicines or balms without a specific description of the constituents:

> For thus saith the Lord:
> Thy hurt is incurable,
> and thy wound is grievous.
> None deemeth of thy wound that
> it may be bound up;
> Thou hast no healing medicines.
> (Jeremiah 30:12, 13)

Jeremiah, prophesying in the 7th century B.C., also speaks of medicines and balms, clearly giving his preference to the latter when he mockingly calls out to Egypt, mortally wounded in battle:

> Go up into Gilead, and take balm,
> O virgin daughter of Egypt;[2]
> In vain dost thou use many medicines;
> There is no cure for thee.
> (Jeremiah 46:11)

In view of the strict hygiene of the ancient Israelites, it is understandable that water should be given first place as a medicine for internal use and in the form of washings and baths. In Leviticus, the Lord repeatedly commands that linen and bedcovers infected by a sick person should be washed. It is clear from the complaint of the sons of the prophets of Jericho to Elisha that fresh water was held in the highest regard: ". . . Behold, we pray thee, the situation of this city is pleasant . . . but the water is bad . . ." (II Kings 2:19) Elisha improves it by performing one of his miracles:

> And he went forth unto the spring of the waters, and cast salt therein, and said: 'Thus saith the Lord: I have healed these waters; there shall not be from thence any more death or miscarrying.'
> (II Kings 2:21)

Biblical people were always quick to take alcoholic drinks prepared by fermenting a variety of raw materials, such as wine from grapes and dates, the latter as a purgative. Vinegar, the oxide product of wine, was also prepared, and when mixed with oil and other ingredients it was used medicinally. Various kinds of oil were applied both internally and externally. A relatively large number of vegetable and animal substances had both a medicinal and a household use. Many of these were used for the same purpose and will be described separately. For example, honey was very popular, and fishgall was a well-known eye remedy.

Pain-killing drugs and smoking also appear as medicinal remedies, while the favorable effect of music on the

---

[2]The "daughter of Egypt" signifies here the Egyptian people.

mentally deranged was well known, an example being David playing on the zither to Saul.

Apothecaries

Those who in the ancient lands of the East were occupied with the preparation of fragrant oils, balms, perfumes, herbal mixtures and spices can be seen as precursors of the present-day apothecaries. In his Bible translation, Luther repeatedly refers to the "apothecary," whereas other translations use the term "perfumer." In Hebrew, *rokeach* literally translates to "the perfumer of ointment," thus "the one who mixes oil with herbs." Modern dispensers can regard the biblical apothecary as a colleague and one who understood his trade very well:

> And Asa [a king] slept with his fathers... and laid him in the bed which was filled with sweet odours and divers kinds [of spices] prepared by the perfumers' art...
> (II Chronicles 16:13, 14)

The perfumer is also mentioned earlier in Exodus when the Lord instructs Moses to make holy anointing oil and perfume:

> 'Take thou also unto thee the chief spices, of flowing myrrh five hundred shekels, and of sweet cinnamon half so much, even two hundred and fifty, and of sweet calamus two hundred and fifty, and of cassia five hundred, after the shekel of the sanctuary, and of olive oil a hin. And thou shalt make it a holy anointing oil, a perfume compounded after the art of the perfumer; it shall be a holy anointing oil.... Take unto thee sweet spices, stacte, and onycha, and galbanum; sweet spices with pure frankincense; of each shall there be a like weight. And thou shalt make of it incense, a

perfume after the art of the perfumer, seasoned with salt, pure and holy.'[3]
(Exodus 30:23-25, 34, 35)

It is evident from the following prohibition to prepare this perfume for private use that this mixture must have been very special:

'. . . it is holy, and it shall be holy unto you. Whosoever compoundeth any like it, or whosoever putteth any of it upon a stranger, he shall be cut off from his people.'
(Exodus 30:32, 33)

From the quantities used to prepare the holy anointing oil, it appears that the oil was not mixed with finely powdered herbs but that the herbs were extracted according to tradition by soaking in water, after which the extract was boiled with the oil.

That the work of apothecaries, or perfumers, was then, as now, usually done by women may be concluded from I Samuel 8:13, where the rights of a king include his taking daughters (of the people) as "confectionaries." The King James version of the Bible uses this translation. The New English Bible uses the word "perfumers" with "confectioners" used as an alternative word.

The perfumer had to ensure that the mixtures were suitably stored. This is pointed out by a lesson from Ecclesiastes:

The words of the wise spoken in quiet
Are more acceptable than the cry of a ruler among
  fools.
Wisdom is better than weapons of war;
But one sinner destroyeth much good.
Dead flies make the ointment of the perfumer
  fetid and putrid . . .
(Ecclesiastes 9:17-10:1)

---

[3] A hin is 6½ liters and a shekel is approximately 16.37 grams; so, 1,500 times 16 grams of spices were used for this balm.

It is quite clear that suitable preparation and storage of spice mixtures entailed accommodations to be used exclusively for the purpose, i.e., housing of the equipment, which could only be used for that purpose. Wealthy Israelites set a room apart to this end, so that a kind of "court dispensary" was attached to the royal palace. King Hezekiah, who lived approximately 700 B.C., permitted the envoys from the King of Babylon to see "all his treasure-house, the silver, and the gold, and the spices and the precious oil . . ." (II Kings 20:13)

A number of utensils, still used in dispensaries, would also have been available in Israel, although the form may slightly differ from what is used today. Infusions and decoctions of fresh and dried herbs were also prepared in those days, and tinctures and vinegars were well known. A licking-pot was prepared from oil and honey; powders were ground in mortars and then put through a sieve. The quality was influenced by the murmur of the words *harik hatif* ("rub finely"). Ointments were frequently used, especially for the eyes or for cosmetic purposes. It is evident from the metaphorical passage in the book of Job that cauldrons were used to boil the ointments:

> He maketh the deep to boil like a pot;
> He maketh the sea like a pot of ointment.
> (Job 41:31)[4]

They had balances with equal arms and two scales, and unequal arms with one scale and a tray, and both metal and stone weights.

The perfumers of antiquity apparently had a guild, as indicated in Nehemiah 3:8: "Hananiah one of the perfumers," helped to rebuild the gates and walls of Jerusalem. A guild must therefore have been in existence by 433 B.C. when Nehemiah, governor of Judah, had the walls of Jerusalem rebuilt.

---

[4]This translation is from the King James Version of the Bible. The New English version also uses the word "ointment." The Masoretic text translates "ointment" as "mixture" (see Job 41:23 in the Masoretic text).

In Ecclesiasticus, a connection is made for the first time between the physician and the apothecary:

> The Lord has created medicines from the earth,
> and a sensible man will not disparage them.
> Was it not a tree that sweetened water
> and so disclosed its properties?
> The Lord has imparted knowledge to men,
> that by their use of his marvels he may win praise;
> by using them the doctor relieves pain
> and from them the pharmacist makes up his mixture.
> There is no end to the works of the Lord,
> who spreads health over the whole world.
> (Ecclesiasticus 38:4-8)

Jesus, son of Sirach, may well have connected both professions with one person, but he nevertheless still made a distinction in the art requisite for the practice of both trades. The physicians who prepared medicine owned an apothecary's chest in which they kept their medicines; it also served as a dispensing table. The flat top was covered with tightly stretched linen or leather on which the plasters were spread after being softened over a fire. The mixture was prepared from oil, wax and resin.

Druggists

Dealers specializing in drugs and related articles are not mentioned in the Bible. But there can be no doubt that modern druggists had forerunners in the land of the ancient Hebrews. Mention is made several times of merchants who carried drugs and spices, and such dealers undoubtedly had fixed dwellings where they stored their goods. The merchants to whom Joseph was sold by his brothers were druggists such as these:

... and, behold, a caravan of Ishmaelites came from Gilead, with their camels bearing spicery and balm and ladanum, going to carry it down to Egypt.

(Genesis 37:25)

Present-day descriptions of travel in the mountainous regions of Palestine give the impression that the country's flora can in no way be described as extraordinary. However, the presence of a wide variety of plants which grew in Europe in early times and which can still be found indicates that the Middle East must be very fertile and that efficient tillage could make ancient Israel a very rich land once again. Greek and Roman writers testify to the flourishing appearance of ancient Palestine, which is further supported by references in the Old Testament:

> And the Lord said: 'I have surely seen the affliction of My people that are in Egypt, and have heard their cry by reason of their taskmasters; for I know their pains; and I am come down to deliver them out of the hand of the Egyptians, and to bring them up out of that land unto a good land and a large, unto a land flowing with milk and honey...'
>
> (Exodus 3:7, 8)

This praise for the land of Israel is repeated in several places, indicating that these words were not prompted by a casual glance on the part of the author of Exodus, but that rich harvests could still be enjoyed by those who would industriously work the soil.

Not all plants referred to in the Bible will be enumerated here. Only those once used medicinally or those still utilized as such belong in this discussion. The words of Sirach have been taken to heart throughout the ages:

> "The Lord has created medicines from the earth,
> and a sensible man will not disparage them."
>
> (Ecclesiasticus 38:4)

It is not always possible to identify with any certainty which plant is indicated from the name or description of a part of a plant given in the Bible. In this respect it resembles the description of illnesses, although the external characteristics of the flowers and leaves give rise to more accurate observation. If the name given is based on pure conjecture, or if it appears that a particular plant is referred to be the general name of an herb, plant, etc., this will be indicated wherever possible.

Roots, Rootstocks, Tubers and Bulbs

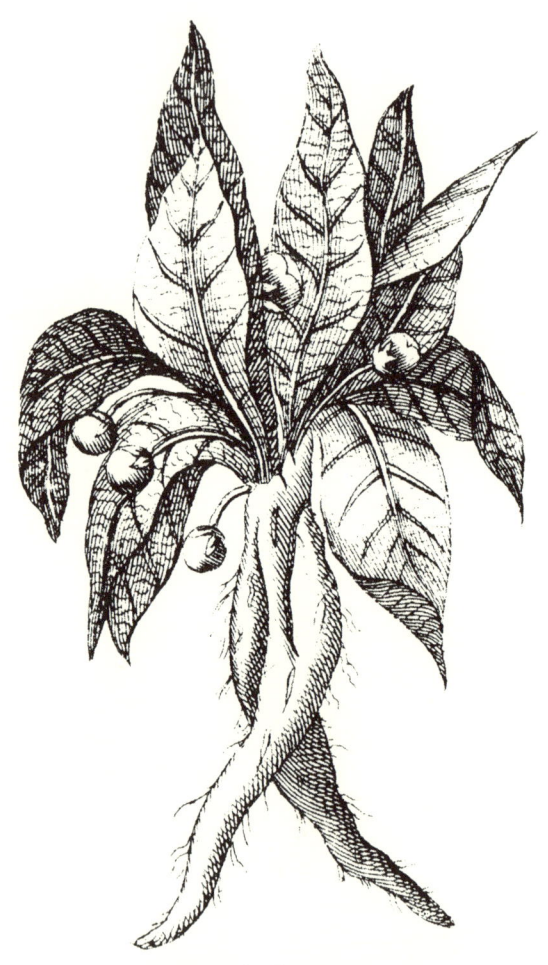

Mandrake Root

Mandrake Root

Atropa mandragora, related to our Deadly Nightshade, belonging to the family of *Solanaceae,* is very common in Palestine and the neighboring countries. This plant has hardly any stem; the leaves and flowers grow close to the root. The latter is shaped like a turnip, sometimes four feet long, a drab brown color on the outside. The figure of a man used to be cut from this root for use in magic. The root itself often has the form of a man; this led to its being called the "Mandrake Man." Love potions prepared from it were said to have the power of fertility. The same effect is also attributed to the yellow berries, *dudaim,* which the plant bears. This probably gave the plant its Hebrew name which is derived from a word meaning "love." It was for this reason that Rachel asked Leah for these berries;

> And Reuben went in the days of wheat harvest, and found mandrakes in the field, and brought them unto his mother Leah. Then Rachel said to Leah: 'Give me, I pray thee, of thy son's mandrakes.' And she said unto her: 'Is it a small matter that thou hast taken away my husband? and wouldest thou take away my son's mandrakes also?'
>
> (Genesis 30:14, 15)

Leah eventually gave away a few of the berries. The story does not relate whether Joseph owes his existence to them. In the Song of Songs, the bridegroom speaks of this plant to his bride with the same purpose in mind when he invites her to join him in a pleasant walk outside:

> ... There will I give thee my love.
> The mandrakes give forth fragrance ...
> (Song of Songs 7:13, 14)

Spiny Restharrow Root

Spiny restharrow root comes from *Ononis spinosa,* a low, thorny shrub which blooms with pink flowers and belongs to the family of *Papilionaceae* and may be found throughout Europe. This "spina" is supposed to be one of the many thorn bushes referred to in several parts of the Old Testament. It is also possible that the Bible refers to a southern European variety: *Ononis antiquorem,* with smaller flowers and leaves but with thorns which are, on the contrary, much longer and stronger. We know for certain that the root rind of this shrub served as a remedy in ancient Greece for kidney stones and was most probably used as such in Palestine. After the Fall of Man, the Lord brings thorns to the earth:

> '... Because thou hast hearkened unto the voice of thy wife, and hast eaten of the tree, of which I commanded thee, saying: Thou shalt not eat of it; cursed is the ground for thy sake; in toil shalt thou eat of it all the days of thy life. Thorns also and thistles shall it bring forth to thee ...'
> (Genesis 3:17, 18)

When Isaiah somberly prophesies the coming of Egyptians and Assyrians to Judah, he describes the wretched state to which they will bring the land, whereby everything will be overgrown with thorns and thistles:

> And it shall come to pass in that day, that every place, where there were a thousand vines at a thousand silverlings, shall even be for briers and thorns. With arrows and with bow shall one come

thither; because all the land shall become briers and thorns. And all the hills that were digged with the mattock, thou shalt not come thither for fear of briers and thorns . . .
(Isaiah 7:23-25)

Thorn branches were also used as birches, perhaps to scourge people to death. Gideon used them to punish the princes and elders of Succoth who had refused to feed his hungry troops on his march against the Midianite kings Zebah and Zalmunna:

> And he took the elders of the city, and thorns of the wilderness and briers, and with them he taught the men of Succoth.
> (Judges 8:16)

There is also metaphorical use made of the thorns in many parts of the Holy Scriptures; for example, in one of the few Old Testament parables that Jotham tells to the Sechemites in order to explain to them that only an unworthy man such as Abimelech will be considered for the position of king. Jotham's story went thus:

> The trees went forth on a time to anoint a king over them; and they said unto the olive-tree: Reign thou over us. But the olive-tree said unto them: Should I leave my fatness, seeing that by me they honour God and man, and go to hold sway over the trees? And the trees said to the fig-tree: Come thou, and reign over us. But the fig-tree said unto them: Should I leave my sweetness, and my good fruitage, and go to hold sway over the trees? And the trees said unto the vine: Come thou, and reign over us. And the vine said unto them: Should I leave my wine, which cheereth God and man, and go to hold sway over the trees? Then said all the trees unto the bramble: Come thou, and reign over us.
> (Judges 9:8-14)

And the thornbush accepted the kingship.

The well-known thorn in the eye can be found in Numbers, the fourth book of Moses. According to the Lord, the Canaanites who are not driven out of Canaan will be a perpetual source of trouble to the Israelites:

> But if ye will not drive out the inhabitants of the land from before you, then shall those that ye let remain of them be as thorns in your eyes, and as pricks in your sides, and they shall harass you in the land wherein ye dwell.
> (Numbers 33:55)

And finally, as one might expect, the thornbush is used metaphorically by the bridegroom in The Song of Songs as a strong contrast with a beautiful flower, his bride:

> As a lily among thorns,
> So is my love among the daughters.
> (The Song of Songs 2:2)

In the Hebrew text, the words *chedek, kotz* and *kimmeshonim* are used for different kinds of thornbush. There are many plants with thorns to be found in Palestine. The "Crown of Thorns" seems to have been made from *Zizyphus spina Christi,* which forms impenetrable hedges and is found abundantly in the Jordan river basin and along the Red Sea: "and plaiting a crown of thorns they placed it on his head..." (Matthew 27:29)

The *Zizyphus* varieties belong to the family of *Rhamnaceae.* A number of other plants, which we shall deal with later in connection with medicinal products, must also be grouped with these thorns—for example: *Capparis spinosa, Astragalus* and *Acacia.*

Broom Root

In the ancient lands of the East, a very bitter broom root, probably derived from *Genista raetem,* seems to have been used medicinally. This plant has white flowers and should not be confused with well-known broom heather which has yellow flowers, but is closely related to it. The herb of *Genista scoparia Lamk,* or *Spartium scoparium L. (Serothamnus scoparius),* which is very common in Europe, is now a depurative folk remedy. It is dangerous to use because of the poisonous alkaloid sparteine. The root of *Genista raetem,* however, does not appear to have been poisonous; in Job there is reference that it is used as a food. Complaining that the people who are far inferior to him deride him in his affliction, Job says:

> They are gaunt with want and famine;
> They gnaw the dry ground . . .
> And the roots of the broom are their food.
> (Job 30:3, 4)

Broom is particularly common in southern Palestine, where it grows alongside rivulets. The shrub has few leaves, but its many branches offer some protection against the sun and wind and it is therefore of great value on bare plains. Elijah, threatened with death by Jezebel, fled to the desert: ". . . and came and sat down under a broom-tree;[5] and he requested for himself that he might die . . ." (I Kings 19:4) Broom charcoal apparently glows for a long time and for this reason was also used to keep a fire burning.

The edibility of this root belonging to the *Papilionaceae* family has possibly been confused with that of *Cynomorium coccineum,* belonging to the *Balanophoraceae* family. The latter lives parasitically on the roots of other plants and is native to all tropical parts of the world. *Cynomorium coccineum* is fleshy and was originally known as *fungus melitensis* and is found in the neighborhood of the Dead Sea. This parasite, or a closely related variety, is still frequently eaten in times of want on the Canary Islands.

---

[5] The King James Version of the Bible translates this as "Juniper tree."

Alkanna Root

The alkanna root was used by ancient West Asiatic people and provided a yellow dye. From this fact it is immediately evident that this plant is not the *Alkanna tinctoria* known to us, with roots that contain the red resinous dye alkannine. This dye, which can be dissolved in alcohol or oil, gives such an intense red color that 1000 to 2000 parts of oil mixed with only one part of alkannine gives a good red tint; so there can be no possibility of confusion with a yellow color. The yellow alkanna root dye used by the ancient Hebrews is given less prominence than the beautiful orange-red dye provided by the leaves of the same plant. These leaves, known under the name of henna, were powdered and boiled in water. From earliest times, eastern women have used this dye to color their nails and hair red. Even the soles of the feet and palms of the hands were treated with it, apparently to strengthen the skin. The flowers of the same plant were much loved for their perfume, and it is again the bridegroom from The Song of Songs who, on beholding the bride, is reminded of these fragrant, white, henna flowers:

> My beloved is unto me as a cluster of henna
> In the vineyards of En-gedi.
> (The Song of Songs 1:14)

The root that provides the yellow dye is the true alkanna root of *Lawsonia inermis,* the Tamr-el-Hinna of the Arabs, belonging to the family of *Lythraceae,* while the false alkanna root that gives the red dye comes from *Alkanna tinctoria,* belonging to the *Boraginaceae*. This is native to southern Europe and is probably the Anchusa of the ancient Greeks. Both the false alkanna root and the henna leaves were used for skin diseases. Since neither can be said to have much medicinal value, they were probably used for this purpose because the extract was the same color as irritated skin.

Iris Root

Bible translations give "cassia" for the Hebrew *kiddah* (which indeed means cassia, or cinnamon) and for *ketzioth*. It is apparently not possible to ascertain if *ketzioth* is another Hebrew word for cinnamon or whether it means another plant altogether, in particular *Iris florentina*. This originated in the mountainous regions of southern Arabia and penetrated southern Europe during the Middle Ages. There is much to be said for this assumption since it is inconceivable that the ancient inhabitants of the lands of the East, who were so very fond of fragrant herbs, would not have utilized this particularly pleasant rootstock that smelled like violets, especially in view of the fact that the plant particularly attracts attention with its white flowers, its flowerlike stigma and sword-shaped leaves. The fragrance of this root is due to the volatile, buttery iris oil which can be extracted by means of distillation with water vapor. The cassia mentioned in Psalms would have been powdered iris root and is more suitable for this specific purpose as a perfume for the clothes of a king than the somewhat strong-smelling cinnamon:

> Myrrh, and aloes, and cassia are all thy garments;
> Out of ivory palaces stringed instruments have made thee glad.
>
> (Psalms 45:9)

Calamus Root

The creeping rootstock of *Acorus calamus,* belonging to the *Araceae,* was already used in ancient times both for the treatment of gastric complaints and as a spice. This rhizome is still used for the same purposes, thanks to the aromatic, essential oil it contains. Although calamus grows throughout the greater part of Europe and can be found there alongside ditches and ponds, its native country is in fact India, and throughout the ages it has spread over northern Asia and Europe. The volatile oil from the cylindrical, pale brown rootstock was an ingredient of the holy anointing oil. There was evidently little calamus to be found in ancient Israel since several places in the Bible refer to its being brought from other countries. For example, Jeremiah warns the people that the outward signs of worship which, they believe, will put them on a favorable footing with the Lord, do not please their God:

> To what purpose is to Me the frankincense that cometh from Sheba,
> And the sweet cane [or calamus], from a far country?
> Your burnt-offerings are not acceptable,
> Nor your sacrifices pleasing unto Me.
>
> (Jeremiah 6:20)

Preparation of the holy anointing oil is described elsewhere as, "Take thou also unto thee: of sweet calamus two hundred and fifty shekels." The use of the word "sweet" can be taken to mean the sweet-smelling *Andropogon calamus aromaticus,* a variety of grass, commonly found in northwest India, exuding a sweet smell when crushed.

Autumn Crocus Corms

The autumn crocus does not appear to have been recognized as a medicinal remedy in antiquity. The name *colchicum autumnale* already indicates that this poisonous tuberous plant blooms in the autumn when all other meadow flowers have bid farewell. According to De Visser, it is the autumn crocus which is referred to in The Song of Songs where the bride says of herself:

> I am a rose of Sharon,
> A lily of the valleys.
>   (The Song of Songs 2:1)

This white or pale lilac-colored flower is inaccurately called a narcissus or a rose in many translations of the Bible. In the original Hebrew text, a specific flower was indicated in the passage quoted from The Song of Songs; its name has been the cause of a variety of translations. Our lily of the valley, *Convallaria majalis,* did not grow in Palestine and so could not possibly have been the flower in question.

Aconite Root

The tuberous roots of *Aconitum napellus,* or monkshood, a plant from the family of *Ranunculaceae,* was not used by the ancient Hebrews as a medicine; this is not so surprising in view of the fact that such extremely poisonous plants were not considered for medical use in those days. The poisonous nature of this herbaceous plant, which grew wild in the mountainous regions of central Europe and central Asia, was in fact very well known in the centuries before the birth of Christ since it was used to kill criminals. Although this plant has a particularly poisonous nature, it is very popular as a decorative plant because of its beautiful violet flowers. The uppermost petal is shaped like a hood, whence the name "monkshood," in German *Sturnhut* or *Eisenhut.*

Garlic

Bulbs from *Allium sativum* (fam. *Liliaceae*) were a very popular form of food seasoning among the ancient Israelites; it must also have been known in Egypt since the Israelites, continuing their journey through the desert, aroused by the rabble, begin to complain again:

> '. . . Would that we were given flesh to eat! We remember the fish, which we were wont to eat in Egypt for nought; the cucumbers, and the melons,

and the leeks, and the onions, and the garlic; but now our soul is dried away; there is nothing at all; we have nought save this manna to look to.'
(Numbers 11:4-6)

It has been said that the Greeks and Romans found garlic a reeking item of food, and the Israelites, who made great use of it, called it *foetentes*. This does not accord with a statement made by Zornig, who contends that garlic prepared with salt as a sauce was a favorite traditional dish in Greece. The Greeks certainly used it medicinally; it would undoubtedly have put new heart into the soldiers. The ancient Hebrews also ascribed the same stimulating properties to these bulbs and used the cloves containing food reserves for the treatment of melancholy and hypochondria. It was also used in those days as a remedy for worms, and it is now available in drugstores for precisely the same purpose. Garlic's anthelmintic properties are due to the volatile oil it contains.

Onion

The memory of the Egyptian onion also made the Israelites' mouths water in the desert (see Garlic); this is not surprising, since the bulbs of *Allium cepa,* which grow along the banks of the Nile, appear to have an exceptionally delicious flavor, and are still one of the principal foods on the market. This bulbous plant is also a member of the *Liliaceae* family. The onion is considered to have a medicinal use as a heart-strengthening remedy and is still used as a laxative and vermicidal.

Leek

The leek is also mentioned in the passage from Numbers quoted above. (See Garlic.) According to Wunderbar, the leek mentioned in the Bible is *Allium porrum,* the leek we eat today. However, De Visser states that "leek" does not mean *Allium porrum* but *Allium schoenoprasum L.*, or chives, a bulbous plant which grows in Europe and can be found wild alongside ponds. It blooms with pink flowers and is also a member of the *Liliaceae* family. Apart from being a normal item of food, the leek is recommended in the Talmud as a dietary remedy in cases of illness.

WOODS AND BARKS

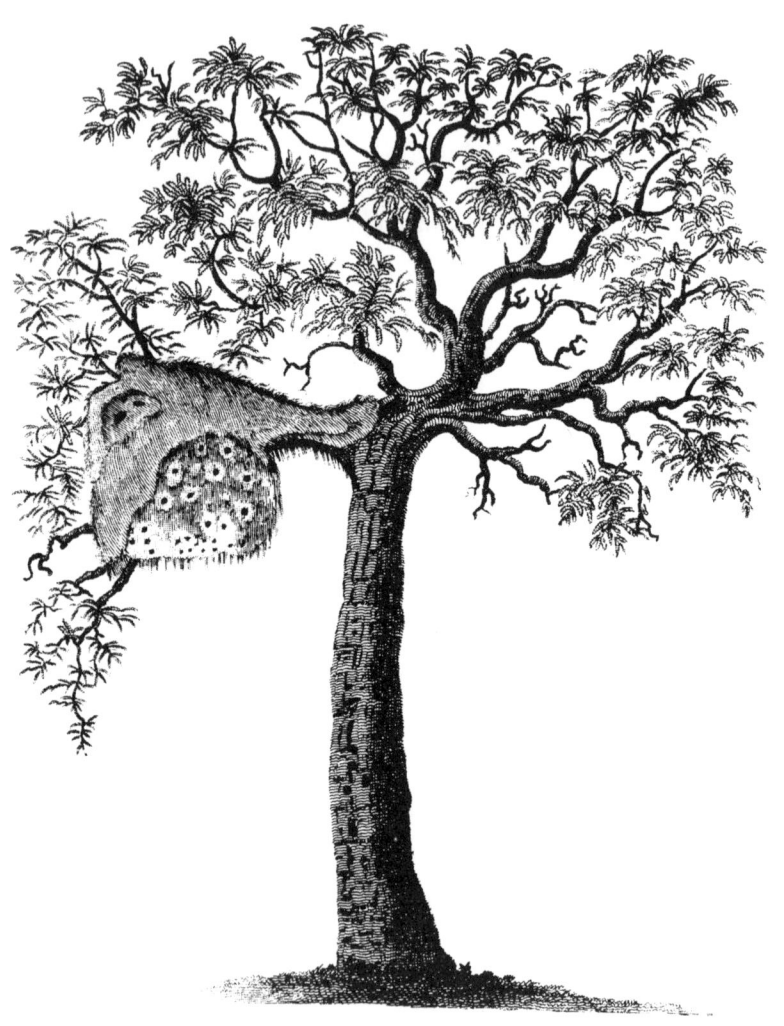

Acacia Tree

Acacia Wood

Of the many varieties belonging to the *Mimosaceae* family native to the whole of tropical Africa, *Acacia arabica Wildd* would have been the wood used for the Ark of the Covenant, the Tabernacle and the sacrificial and incense altars. The acacia tree has dark brown wood that is very light and can be beautifully polished, a factor that makes it suitable for manufacturing all kinds of commodities. The fact that it grew in the desert designated this tree as a supplier of wood:

> And the Lord spoke unto Moses, saying . . . 'And they shall make an ark of acacia-wood . . .'

Even the staves on which this sacred chest was carried were made of the same wood:

> 'And thou shalt make a table of acacia-wood . . . And thou shalt set upon the table showbread before Me alway. And thou shalt make the boards for the tabernacle of acacia-wood, standing up . . . And thou shalt make bars of acacia-wood . . . And thou shalt make the altar of acacia-wood . . .'
> (Exodus 25:1, 10, 30; 26:15, 26; 27:1)

It is evident from the prophecy in Isaiah that different varieties of acacia were also to be found in the promised land. Israel, still in a state of wretchedness, will soon be miraculously blessed by the Lord:

> I will open rivers on the high hills,
> And fountains in the midst of the valleys,
> I will make the wilderness a pool of water,
> And the dry land springs of water.
> I will plant in the wilderness the cedar, the acacia-tree,
> And the myrtle, and the oil-tree;
> I will set in the desert the cypress, the plane-tree, and the larch together . . .
> (Isaiah 41:18, 19)

This tree has great medicinal importance due to its highly valued gum which flows from splits in the bark during the blossoming period. Gum arabic used in pharmacies today does not actually come from *Acacia arabica,* but from *Acacia Senegal.* The name "arabic" is due to the fact that this variety found west of the Nile was brought from Arabia by the Arabs to be traded here and there. Trade in gum is already mentioned in the first book of Moses. Gum, which hardens on contact with air, is sold in the form of yellow round or angular pieces about the size of a marble. It has a faintly slimy taste. The prodigious glueing power of wet gum is applied in the preparation of pastilles (hard candies), for example.

Sandalwood

Red sandalwood was used medicinally by the Arabs; the white wood was held in high esteem by ancient China and India because of its aromatic smell. It is still used in those countries as a perfume in religious proceedings and death cults. Red sandalwood is only slightly aromatic. The hard, dark red wood lends itself better than the white to the manufacture of armrests and musical instruments. The red wood is technically known as caliatour and can be exquisitely polished. In powder form, it serves as a dye for varnish, and is added to toothpowders and ointments by pharmacists for the same purpose. White sandalwood is rather soft and of much greater importance in present-day medicine since it provides the well-known and much used *oleum santali* which is obtained by distillation.

> And when the queen of Sheba heard of the fame of Solomon because of the name of the Lord, she came to prove him with hard questions. And she came to Jerusalem with a very great train, with camels that bore spices and gold very much, and precious stones . . . And the navy also of Hiram, that brought gold from Ophir, brought in from Ophir great plenty of sandal-wood and precious stones. And the kind made of the sandal-wood pillars for the house of the Lord, and for the king's house, harps also and psalteries for the singers; there came no such sandal-wood, nor was seen, unto this day.
> (I Kings 10:1, 2, 11, 12)

The "almug tree" mentioned in this biblical passage could be the type of sandalwood known as *Santalum album,* which produces a white wood. *Pterocarpus santalinus* produces a dark red wood. Both varieties are native to India and were known to the ancient peoples of the East. The land of Ophir mentioned in the passage above is believed to lie either in southern Arabia or India.

Santalum album is an evergreen tree six to seven meters high, with dense foliage, belonging to the family of *Santalaceae*. *Pterocarpus santalinus* is a tree of approximately the same height, but belongs to the family of *Leguminosae.*

Willow Bark

Although it is hardly used at all today for medicinal purposes, the bark of different varieties of willow tree, such as *Salix alba* and *Salix fragilis,* was for a short time used for its salicin, a glucoside which supplies salicylic acid. In ancient times willow twigs were used for basketwork and the bark served as tanning material.

The use of willow as a peg for the lyre is not a recent invention. The singer in Psalms recalls the time when he and his companions sat weeping by the rivers of Babylon and could not sing any songs about Zion, as their enemies desired, since they could never forget Jerusalem:

> By the rivers of Babylon,
> There we sat down, yea, we wept,
> When we remembered Zion.
> Upon the willows in the midst thereof
> We hanged up our harps.
> For there they that led us captive asked of us words
>   of song,
> And our tormentors asked of us mirth . . .
> (Psalms 137:1-3)

The willow indicated here could be the Babylonian or weeping willow, which was brought to Europe from the East: it has also been suggested that the willows mentioned in the Bible were poplars, also members of the *Salicaceae* family. The brook willow is referred to by name in Leviticus 23:40. Branches from these riverside trees must have been merrily waved to celebrate the feast of harvest—a custom also known among the Greeks and Romans.

Oak Bark

Two very important trees in antiquity which should be mentioned in connection with the *simplicia* are the oak and the terebinth. Both of these trees were much sought after for religious worship and are mentioned in Genesis:

> And Abram moved his tent, and came and dwelt
> by the terebinths of Mamre, which are in Hebron,
> and built there an altar unto the Lord . . . And the

Lord appeared unto him by the terebinths of Mamre, as he sat in the tent door in the heat of the day . . .

(Genesis 13:18 and 18:1)

In olden times, the Hebrew words for oak and terebinth were often used synonymously, although "alloon" and "allah" more specifically referred to the oak, while "êl" and "elah" were used to indicate the terebinth.

Different types of oak grow in Palestine. *Quercus infectoria,* native to Asia, grows in the form of a bush. The sting of a gallfly on the young branches causes the formation of gallnuts, or oak apples, which often contain more than 60% tannic acid. These nuts are highly sought after by ink manufacturers since tannic acid produces a fine dark-blue compound with iron.

The *Quercus sessiflora,* the evergreen sessile oak, belonging to the family of *Cupuliferae,* was also found in ancient Israel. This is commonly cultivated today in Europe for its bark, which, thanks to its tannic acid content, is used in leather tanning and was a remedy applied in the dim past for blood-spitting and colic, and is now used as a styptic and astringent.

Cinnamon

The bark of the branches of *Cinnamomum cassia* is the oldest spice mentioned. Cinnamon was already known in China in 2700 B.C., and was used by the Egyptians by 1500 B.C., where Moses learned about its agreeable properties. Fragrant cinnamon happened to be one of the ingredients commanded for the holy anointing oil (Exodus 30:23).

Hebrew *kinnamon* is *Kaju manis* in Malay, meaning sweet root. Although I cannot find this explanation recorded anywhere, I think that Moses used the sticks of cinnamon that he took from Egypt not only for the holy oil, but also to improve the bitter taste of the water of Marah. The Bible states that Moses made the water "sweet"; this naturally leads one to the conclusion that sweet root may have been used. Today, the strongly aromatic *oleum cinnamomi,* obtained from the bark of the branches, is used both for medicinal purposes and to make bitter or otherwise unpleasant medicines palatable. It should be borne in mind that desert water is not so bitter as to be absolutely undrinkable since the Arabs and their camels drink it if better water is unavailable.

> And Moses led Israel onward from the Red Sea, and they went out into the wilderness of Shur; and they went three days in the wilderness, and found no water. And when they came to Marah, they could not drink of the waters of Marah, for they were bitter. Therefore the name of it was called Marah. And the people murmured against Moses, saying: 'What shall we drink?' And he cried unto the Lord; and the Lord showed him a tree, and he cast it into the waters, and the waters were made sweet . . .
> (Exodus 15:22-25)

Hardly any plants grow in Marah; only the dates from the date palms growing there could have sweetened the water somewhat. But it seems quite feasible that Moses used the sticks of cinnamon he had brought from Egypt.

This treelike plant from the *Lauraceae* family is grown in many tropical countries today. The outer layer of the branch bark, which is whitish or gray and almost tasteless and scentless, is removed; the inner rind is marketed in curled strips. In the places where the Bible speaks of cassia, cinnamon is generally indicated, although the same word may refer to iris root.

Gossypium Bark

An extract from the root bark of *Gossypium herbaceum,* the cotton plant, is currently used medicinally as a styptic. The light brown cortex is exported to Europe from North America. People in the ancient world were not aware of its medicinal property, but they certainly knew the plant itself. Two varieties, *Gossypium religiosum* and *Gossypium hirsutum,* were cultivated in the earliest times in the East Indies and Arabia, in order to obtain the cotton, in the form of yellow-colored pappus or fiber, which is found when the fruit bursts open. This exceptionally useful shrub, belonging to the family of *Malvaceae,* even flourishes in poor soil. In 1000 B.C., cotton had spread from India to Babylon and Egypt, then later to Greece. It was woven into the finest cloth; the Egyptians and the Israelites (following their stay in Egypt) soon began to cultivate the plants. The fiber, 2-4 centimeters long, contains a considerable amount of oil which first has to be removed; after further cleaning, pure cotton wool is obtained.

Clothes made of cotton were very expensive in the time of the Hebrews, and were only to be worn by rich or important people. The Hebrew word for cotton is *sjeesj.* Like the words *boes* and *bad,* this word indicated vegetable matter as opposed to wool. In many cases the Bible refers to linen where it means cotton, and vice versa. Luther even refers to "silk."

It appears from Exodus that cotton was highly valued since the Lord demanded it as a gift for himself:

> And the Lord spoke unto Moses, saying: 'Speak unto the children of Israel, that they take for Me an offering; of every man whose heart maketh him willing ye shall take My offering. And this is the offering which ye shall take of them: gold, and silver, and brass; and blue, and purple, and

scarlet, and fine linen, and goats' hair; and rams' skins dyed red, and sealskins, and acacia-wood; oil for the light, spices for the anointing oil, and for the sweet incense; onyx stones, and stones to be set, for the ephod, and for the breastplate.'
(Exodus 25:1-7)

Of these gifts for the furnishing of the sanctuary, only cotton is mentioned for the drapery, and this was also the material used for the priestly vestments: "And they shall make the ephod of gold, of blue, and purple, scarlet, and fine twined linen, the work of skilful workman." (Exodus 28:6) It is not clear whether the yellow-colored cotton was completely dyed with the forementioned dyes, or whether only the figures woven into the cloth were colored.

Pomegranate Bark

The fame of the pomegranate tree is due to its fruit, the pomegranate, which has a brilliant scarlet-red peel. In The Song of Songs, the cheeks of the bride are compared with the juicy red pulp:

Thy lips are like a thread of scarlet,
And thy mouth is comely;
Thy temples are like a pomegranate split open
Behind thy veil.
(The Song of Songs 4:3)

Since the flowers are also a brilliant, pure red, this tree in blossom is a wonderful sight and is often grown as a decorative plant. Possibly because of its large number of pips, the pomegranate was a symbol of fertility for some nations. In Israel, the image of a pomegranate was a decorative motif for sacred objects (I Kings 7:18). I have, however, been unable to find a single passage in the Bible where mention is made of the pomegranate's use as a medicine. The rather sour pulp was certainly used to prepare refreshing drinks and the rind was employed to tan and color Moroccan leather. The bride in The Song of Songs wishes to refresh her beloved with this must:

> ... I would cause thee to drink of spiced wine,
> Of the juice of my pomegranate.
> (The Song of Songs 8:2)

Both the root and the stem rind as well as the peel of the pomegranate are now used medicinally; the root and bark as a vermicidal and the peel for its astringent properties. *Punica granatum* belongs to the family of *Punicaceae,* and is commonly cultivated in southern Europe and tropical regions.

Herbs, Leaves, Leaf-Buds, Flowers and Parts of Flowers

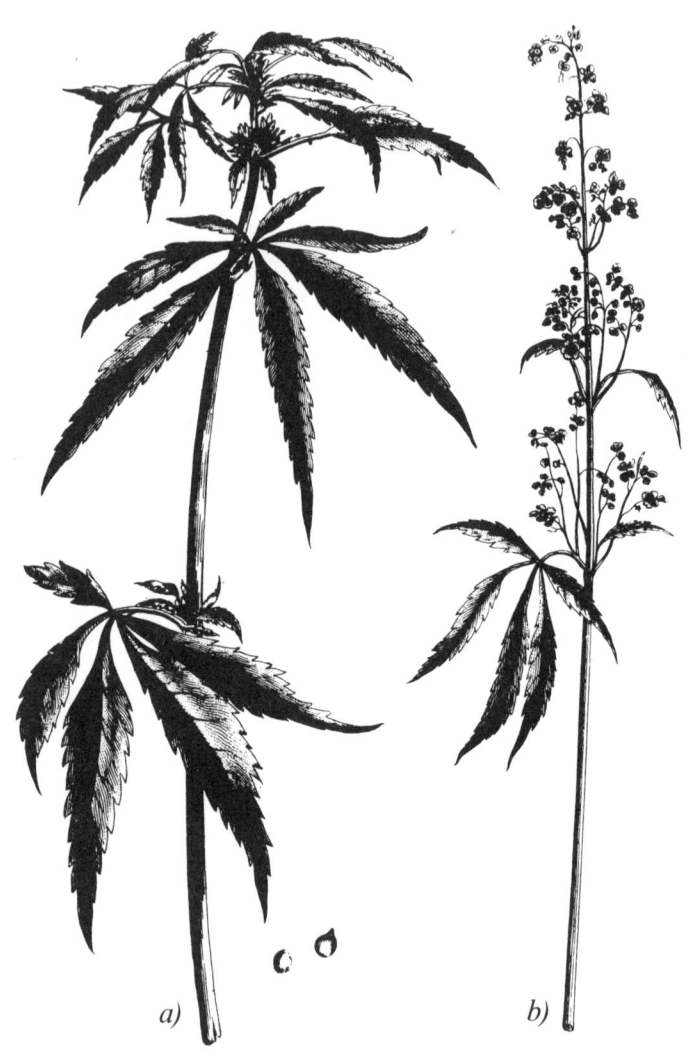

Indian Hemp
a) female; b) male. Note that the female hemp is the Bible reference.

Sabine

This is "heath" or common heather, a term which principally covers plants belonging to the *Ericaceae* family. Of the many plants belonging to this group, only a few varieties are found in Syria, but these do not grow in the desert. Since the Arabic word for "juniper" is the same as the Hebrew word for "heather," and both *Juniperus sabina* and *Juniperus communis* belong to the family of *Coniferae,* native to the desert and bare, rocky regions of Syria, they are probably the "heather" referred to in the Bible. Sabine herb is an evergreen shrub which is cultivated in Europe. Its leaves are believed to be an abortifacient. The ancient Sabines apparently used these needle-shaped leaves for this purpose. An essential oil is the active ingredient.[6]

Jeremiah prophesies misery for whomever puts his trust in men and not in the Lord: "For he shall be like the heath in the desert..." (Jeremiah 17:6)[7] Further on, where the Lord portends the ruin of the cities of Moab, the people are advised to flee. General misery will, however, still follow:

> Flee, save your lives,
> And be like the heath in the wilderness.
> (Jeremiah 48:6)[8]

---

[6] For *Juniperus communis* see Juniper Fruit, page 60.
[7] This translation is from the King James version of the Bible.
[8] This translation is from the King James version of the Bible.

Indian Hemp

The narcotic variety of *Cannabis sativa,* belonging to the family of *Cannabinaceae,* plays a major role as an anesthetic and narcotic remedies among Asiatic and African tribes. Both the herb of the female plant and the resin (released from glands on the branches and leaves) are used. It is prepared in several different ways and may be smoked, chewed, eaten or drunk. The narcotic effect was known in 800 B.C. in China and Asia. The extract drawn from this herb is still used medicinally as, among other things, a painkiller in corn ointment or plasters. Fabric from hemp fiber was used by the ancient Israelites for clothing, but was later replaced for this purpose by cotton and linen. It was more often cultivated for its strong fibers and hemp seed, used in carpets and in rope. The latter was used in the days of Moses for making the sanctuary:

> 'And let every wise-hearted man among you come, and make all that the Lord hath commanded... the hangings of the court, the pillars thereof, and their sockets, and the screen for the gate of the court; the pins of the tabernacle, and the pins of the court, and their cords...'
> (Exodus 35:10, 17, 18)

Stinging Nettle

It is not possible to ascertain which type of plant is indicated when the word "nettles" is used in the Bible, although references to special stinging nettles do occur. For example, when Job is taunted by the inferior people, he compares them to asses and says:

> Among the bushes they bray;
> Under the nettles they are gathered together.
> (Job 30:7)

The "small nettle" *(Urtica urens)*, now used in homeopathy to stimulate milk production, and *Urtica dioica* (stinging nettle), from the *Urticaceae* family, can be included with these nettles since they are both native to Palestine.

Greater Celandine

The yellow sap this herb contains has a nauseating smell and a bitter taste. The fresh sap is commonly used for smearing on warts and freckles, while the extract is employed for the treatment of cancer. In antiquity, the herb was used for eye complaints and jaundice; this was probably due to the similarity in color of the golden-yellow root. This color later inspired the alchemists to use the root for their gold-making activities; they also said that the name *chelidonium* was derived from *celi (caeli)*, meaning heaven, and *doneum*, or gift. The plant's name is actually the Greek *chelidon*, meaning "swallow," since the plant blooms in Europe during the whole period that the swallows are there.

Rue

This dried herb is used exclusively as a folk remedy. In ancient times it was considered an important medicine, as indicated by the name *ruta*, from a Greek word meaning "to save." The herb was particularly popular as an antiseptic since the volatile oil was believed to expel all bad matter. When gathered before the plant blooms, the leaves have a strong, even unpleasant smell; when the plant has been dried, the smell is milder. *Ruta graveolene* is one of the many types belonging to the family of *Rutaceae* which are native to the region around the Mediterranean Sea. The leaves were also a favorite culinary herb. The plant was cultivated for this purpose and as such was taxed, as is evident from Jesus' answer to the Pharisees who marveled that the Lord had not first washed before the midday meal:

> But the Lord said to him, 'You Pharisees! You clean the outside of cup and plate; but inside you there is nothing but greed and wickedness. . . . Alas for you Pharisees! You pay tithes of mint and rue and every garden-herb, but have no care for justice and the love of God. It is these you should have practised, without neglecting the others.'
> (Luke 11:39, 42)

Hemlock

The prophet Hosea prophesies that Israel will still have to endure much suffering for its pride and wantonness, that even their king will be of no avail:

> Surely now shall they say:
> 'We have no king;
> For we feared not the Lord;
> And the king, what can he do for us?'
> They speak words,
> They swear falsely, they make covenants;
> Thus judgment springeth up as hemlock
> In the furrows of the field.
> (Hosea 10:3, 4)

The word hemlock *(Conium maculatum)* is the translation given here for the Hebrew *rosh*. This umbelliferous plant can now be found as a weed all over the world, but originally it only grew in Asia. Its poisonous property, caused by the liquid alkaloid coniine, was well known in ancient times, and the hemlock drink to which Socrates was condemned was prepared from this herb. Hemlock is recognizable by the red speckles all over the lower part of the hollow stem.

The Greek word *conium* means "stimulating dizziness," referring thus to its effect. Hemlock is still used medicinally to relieve pain and cramp.

Hyssop

When celebrating a number of cleansing rites, the ancient Israelites used hyssop for sprinkling. The leaves quickly absorb moisture and, when they are shaken, release it again:

> Then Moses called for all the elders of Israel, and said unto them: 'Draw out, and take you lambs according to your families, and kill the passover lamb. And ye shall take a bunch of hyssop, and dip it in the blood that is in the basin, and strike the lintel and the two side-posts with the blood that is in the basin; and none of you shall go out of the door of his house until the morning.
> (Exodus 12:21, 22)

Hyssop was also used for the ritual cleansing of a leper:

> And the Lord spoke unto Moses, saying: This shall be the law of the leper in the day of his cleansing: he shall be brought unto the priest. And the priest shall go forth out of the camp; and the priest shall look, and, behold, if the plague of leprosy be healed in the leper; then shall the priest command to take for him that is to be cleansed two living clean birds, and cedar-wood, and scarlet, and hyssop.
> (Leviticus 14:1-4)

The hyssop is dipped in the blood of one of the birds and the leper is sprinkled with it seven times. The Roman Catholic church still refers to the hyssop holy water sprinkler.

Never has there been so much divided opinion over a biblical herb as that over hyssop. *Hyssopus officinalis,* a branched shrub belonging to the family of *Labiatae,* grown in European gardens for culinary purposes, is apparently not identical with the Hebrew *esob,* the holy herb. The labiate mentioned above did not occur in Asia Minor. The wisdom of Solomon gives us some hint. He speaks "of trees, from the cedar that is in Lebanon even unto the hyssop that springeth out of the wall. . ." (I Kings 5:13)[9] But there are numerous plants which grow on walls. One may conclude from this, however, that the sacred herb was not a large plant. There is much to be said for the contention that the "hyssop" of antiquity was *Capparis spinosa* (see Capers in this section) which grows in abundance on the walls of Jerusalem, is commonly found on dry, stony places and also in the desert, since Moses fetched this plant from the desert for the feast of the Passover.

Another opinion is that the biblical hyssop comes from *Origanum aegypticum,* a kind of marjoram, the only labiate which was native to the East. Further confusion arises from the fact that the Gospel of John states: ". . . and they filled a sponge with vinegar, and put it upon hyssop, and put it to his mouth." (John 19:29)[10]

But St. Matthew claims that a sponge filled with vinegar was put on a "reed" (Matthew 27:48) so as to give Jesus a drink before his death. Comparing "put . . . upon hyssop" with "a reed," one must conclude that hyssop was a shrub with branches long enough to be able to reach the mouth of Jesus. It is conceivable that the sponge was placed on a bunch of hyssop, transfixed on a reed. This explanation would bring the hyssop back to a low, herbaceous plant. *Hyssopus officinalis* was sporadically used for medicinal purposes as an expectorant and an antirheumatic remedy, the latter more as a folk remedy.

---

[9]The reader should note that this is I Kings 4:33 in the King James Version of the Bible.
[10]This translation is from the King James version of the Bible.

Common Wormwood Flower Heads

Common wormwood is one of the oldest remedies and was known as such in Egypt in 1600 B.C. *Artemisia absinthium* was native to southern and central Europe and in western and northern Asia. The common name wormwood indicates its use; it was a favorite for cattle in particular.

The flower heads of wormwood (family *Compositae*) contain the hallucinogen santonin, a volatile oil, and a bitter principle, absinthiine. The raceme-shaped inflorescences are used in liqueur distillation for the preparation of absinthe which, when drunk to excess, has a damaging effect and causes delirium. The essential oil is a green color to which absinthe owes its famous appearance. The German "wermut" also apparently refers to its vermicidal property (vermes = worm).

The intensely bitter taste of wormwood gave the authors of the Bible many opportunities to compare it with the unpleasant aspects of life. A warning is given in Proverbs about relations with strange women which lead to ruin:

> For the lips of a strange woman drop honey,
> And her mouth is smoother than oil;
> But her end is bitter as wormwood,
> Sharp as a two-edged sword.
> (Proverbs 5:3, 4)

It is evident from the punishment given by the Lord to false prophets that wormwood is considered to be very disagreeable:

> Behold, I will feed them with wormwood,
> And make them drink the water of gall;
> For from the prophets of Jerusalem
> Is ungodliness gone forth into all the land.
> (Jeremiah 23:15)

Poplar Buds

The poplar tree belongs to the same family as the willow (see Willow Bark, page 33). *Gemmae populi,* which come from different varieties of *populus,* are yellow-brown, sticky, bullet-shaped leaf buds which are gathered before budding. A tincture of these buds is used in an ointment. *Populus nigra* is native to Asia and was commonly found along the eastern bank of the Jordan, opposite Jericho. Jacob used poplar wood to increase his possessions after Laban had agreed that Jacob might have every speckled and spotted animal in the flock.

> And Jacob took him rods of fresh poplar, and of the almond and of the plane-tree; and peeled white streaks in them, making the white appear which was in the rods. And he set the rods which he had peeled over against the flocks in the gutters in the watering-troughs where the flocks came to drink; and they conceived when they came to drink. And the flocks conceived at the sight of the rods, and the flocks brought forth streaked, speckled, and spotted.
>
> (Genesis 30:37-39)

Walnut Leaves

Although there is no direct reference to the walnut tree in the Bible, it is certainly indirectly mentioned in The Song of Songs where there is an allusion to the "garden of nuts":

> I went down into the garden of nuts,
> To look at the green plants of the valley,
> To see whether the vine budded,
> And the pomegranates were in flower.
> (The Song of Songs 6:11)

The reference is undoubtedly to *Juglans regia,* our walnut tree, belonging to the family of *Juglandaceae,* a native to western Asia and the eastern part of the Mediterranean, and which is now grown throughout Europe. Walnut leaves are still used in folk medicine for the treatment of worms and gout.

Laurel Leaves

The leaves and fruit of the *Laurus nobilis,* the laurel, still have their place as a culinary herb and a medicinal remedy. This evergreen tree from the family of *Lauraceae,* which is native to the Mediterranean region, is not specifically referred to by name in the Bible—a surprising fact since the ancient Israelites seasoned their food with herbs and spices and would certainly have been acquainted with the laurel leaf. The laurel may possibly be the tree referred to in Psalms where mention is made of "a leafy tree in its native soil." (Psalms 37:35) [11]

Peppermint Leaves

In Jesus' reply to the Pharisees quoted in this chapter under Rue, he mentioned not only tithes of rue, but also mint. It is impossible to be sure what variety of mint is alluded to. *Mentha* is an extensive genus belonging to the family of *Labiatae.* All are very aromatic. Peppermint and spearmint are both commonly known as culinary and medicinal herbs. The essential oil obtained from the leaves contains menthol, which is used as a particularly cooling remedy in the treatment of migraine. It has been ascertained that

---

[11] In the King James Version, this tree is referred to as "... a green tree that groweth in his own soil."

Mentha piperita was an ancient Chinese plant, and that the Egyptians recognized the medicinal value of this herb in 1550 B.C. The Greeks and Romans learned of it via Palestine.

Bramble Leaves

The delicious fruit of the bramble-berry (blackberry) is still highly valued, even though biblical references hold it in lower regard than the grape. "For each tree is known by its own fruit: you do not gather figs from thistles, and you do not pick grapes from brambles." (Luke 6:44) Appreciation of bramble leaves has considerably lessened throughout the ages. The ancient Arabs utilized them as an aphrodisiac; they were later used medicinally as a diuretic and for the treatment of diarrhea; they are now only a folk remedy. The thorny plant *Rubus fructuosus,* belonging to the *Rosaceae* family, can be found growing wild throughout Europe and Asia.

Saffron

Saffron crocus produces the unusual dark-yellow stigma which can be found in groups of three on the top of the style in the pale violet flowers. The name "saffron" is due to the yellow matter obtained from it. The Arabic word *safra* means "yellow." Apart from the dye, which still has technical and household uses, saffron was held in the highest regard by the ancient Egyptians because of its pleasant, aromatic taste and smell. *Crocus sativus,* of the *Iridaceae* family, is a tuberous plant, native to Asia Minor and the Levant, and is extensively grown in southern Europe, especially Spain. Tinctures of saffron are still used medicinally as gastric and intestinal remedies. The bridegroom in The Song of Songs boasts that his bride is like a garden of Eden full of delightful flowers, including *Crocus sativus:*

> Thy shoots are a park of pomegranates,
> With precious fruits;
> Henna with spikenard plants,
> Spikenard and saffron, calamus and cinnamon,
> With all trees of frankincense;
> Myrrh and aloes, with all the chief spices.
> (The Song of Songs 4:13, 14)

Cloves

Moses possibly included cloves, or "nails," in his holy perfume. The word "clove" is derived from the French *clou,* Latin *clavus,* meaning "a nail." Most versions of the Bible use the word "onycha"[12]: And the Lord said unto Moses: 'Take unto thee sweet spices, stacte, and onycha, and galbanum; sweet spices with pure frankincense...' (Exodus 30:34) Onycha, from the Greek word *onux,* means "nail." What kind of nail is meant is not absolutely clear. Since reference is made to "sweet spices," it may be assumed that onycha is of vegetable origin. In the proverbs of Jesus son of Sirach, the delightful smell of onyx is again mentioned:

> Like cassia or camel-thorn I was redolent of spices;
> I spread my fragrance like choice myrrh,
> like galban, aromatic shell, and gum resin;
> I was like the smoke of incense in the sacred tent.
> (Ecclesiasticus 24:15)

The semiprecious stone onyx has no smell of its own and can therefore be excluded.

---
[12]*The New English Bible* uses "aromatic shell."

What we today refer to as cloves are the flower heads of *Eugenia caryophyllata,* belonging to the family of *Myrtaceae,* native to the Molukken Islands and grown in many tropical countries. It is impossible to ascertain if the ancient Hebrews knew this spice. Before the birth of Christ, the Chinese apparently chewed on cloves. The clove may have spread from China by means of trading, although this is not certain. The name of the flower bud is due to the sometimes 12 mm-long interior ovary. Since the unopened flower is red, the tree in full bloom is an exquisite sight. When dried, the buds turn brown. Cloves are used medicinally as a stomachic. The essential oil also has a technical application.

Caper Buds

The caper is a common bush in Palestine and belongs to the family of *Capparidaceae.* The young flower buds are round, hard and olive green, which is why they are referred to as "caper berries." The flower buds of *Capparis spinosa,* found in southern Europe and the East, were used either raw or drawn in vinegar or date wine to stimulate the appetite; they were also used to stimulate sexual desire. Today their only application is as a folk medicine. Capers are metaphorically referred to in Ecclesiastes in relation to the end of human life:

> Also when they shall be afraid of that which is high,
> And terrors shall be in the way;
> And the almond-tree shall blossom,
> And the grasshopper shall drag itself along,
> And the caperberry shall fail;
> Because man goeth to his long home,
> And the mourners go about the streets. . .
> (Ecclesiastes 12:5)

An alternative translation for "fail" is "burst open," a sign that the caper flower has reached the end of the blooming period.

FRUITS AND SEEDS

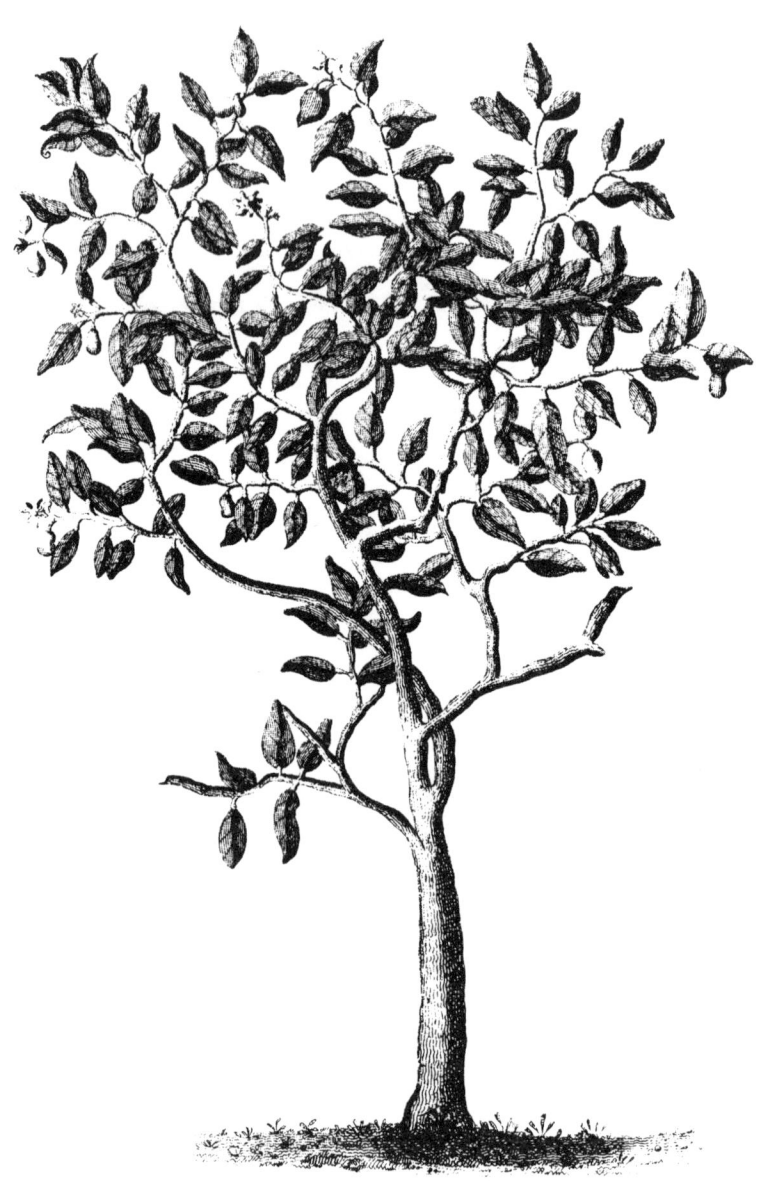

Lemon Tree

Dates

The date palm formerly grew in Palestine, especially in the area around Jericho, which is why the latter was called the "city of palm-trees." ". . . the South, and the Plain, even the valley of Jericho the city of palm-trees, as far as Zoar." (Deuteronomy 34:3) The palm tree, which can attain a height of 100 feet, is rarely found in that particular place today. The fruits, which grow together in a bunch, are red when ripe and are eaten raw; a syrup is prepared from the sap. A date wine is also prepared from the sap, and was used medicinally in ancient times.

The date palm's name, *Phoenix dactylifera,* family *Palmae,* comes from the region of Phoenicia where it was especially common. Dates were an important and a favorite food of the Israelites, and still are for the tribes of Bedouins in the desert:

> And they came to Elim, where were twelve springs of water, and three score and ten palm-trees; and they encamped there by the waters.
> (Exodus 15:27)

Palm branches were used for the Feast of Tabernacles:

> '. . . Go forth unto the mount, and fetch olive branches, and branches of wild olive, and myrtle branches, and palm branches, and branches of thick trees, to make booths, as it is written.'
> (Nehemiah 8:15)

Palm branches are also a sign of respect with which kings are welcomed:

> The next day the great body of pilgrims who had come to the festival, hearing that Jesus was on the way to Jerusalem, took palm branches and went out to meet him, shouting, 'Hosanna! Blessings on him who comes in the name of the Lord! God bless the king of Israel!'
> (John 12:12, 13)

Palm leaves were of major technical significance as they were used to make all kinds of basket work, while the leaf fibers were manufactured into mats and bags.

The date palm has no significance today in the field of medicine. Only the wine prepared from the sap is still used as a stimulant. Indian "arrack" is distilled from this. Palm wine is possibly the "strong drink" referred to in the Bible, for example, in Judges where an angel of the Lord appeared to the wife of Manoah of the Danites, prophesying that she would bear a son (Samson) who would be a "Nazirite unto God": "Now therefore beware, I pray thee, and drink no wine nor strong drink . . ." (Judges 13:4)

Juniper Berries

In the passages where the Dutch Leiden translation of the Bible refers to "Broom," the German translation gives "Wachholder," and the King James version refers to the "Juniper Tree":

> For want and famine they were solitary; fleeing into the wilderness in former time desolate and waste. Who cut up mallows by the bushes, and juniper roots for their meat.
> (Job 30:3, 4)

This is *Juniperus communis,* belonging to the family of *Coniferae,* an evergreen shrub, which grows throughout

Europe, North America and Central Asia. This plant could have grown in Palestine, but the root is not edible, although the root of the broom tree was probably equally inedible. Juniper berries are used in the distillation of gin. The ripe, dark brown, sometimes blue, berries are used medicinally as a stomachic.

Husked Barley

Barley, belonging to the family of *Graminaceae,* is considered to be the oldest kind of grain. The floury kernel of the fruit of *Hordeum vulgare* and *Hordeum distichum* is still used medicinally for its high starch content in the preparation of mealy, viscous medicines.

During one of the plagues of Egypt, the Lord's punishment is to ruin the barley by a hailstorm: "And the flax and the barley were smitten; for the barley was in the ear, and the flax was in bloom." (Exodus 9:31)

It is evident from a passage in Leviticus that barley played an important role as food for both men and beasts. The Law of the Vows determines what must be paid by a man who has dedicated a field to the Lord. The value of this land is estimated in accordance with the quantity of barley needed to sow it:

> And if a man shall sanctify unto the Lord part of the field of his possession, then thy valuation shall be according to the sowing thereof; the sowing of a homer of barley shall be valued at fifty shekels of silver.
> (Leviticus 27:16)

Barley bread was among the masses in the time of Jesus. The Lord used it to feed the multitude who had followed him over the Sea of Galilee: "There is boy here who has five barley loaves and two fishes; but what is that among so many?" (John 6:9) By performing one of his miracles, Jesus was able to satisfy about 5,000 people with this food.

Poppy Capsules

Although the Bible does not specifically refer by name to the capsules or other parts of the *Papaver somniferum L. (Papaver setigerum DC)*, a few observations should be made about this plant because it has been suggested that the "wine mingled with gall" which was given to Jesus to drink before the crucifixion may have been an acetic acid infusion of poppy seeds.

> So they came to a place called Golgotha (which means 'Place of a skull') and there he was offered a draught of wine mixed with gall; but when he had tasted it he would not drink.
> (Matthew 27:33, 34)

A much more acceptable explanation would be that Jesus, noticing that they were trying to give him a narcotic mixture given to criminals who were crucified to alleviate the pain, refused it so as to die fully conscious rather than that he was deterred by the bitter taste of the fish or animal gall. In Psalms 69:21 the word gall can also be found.[13] It should be mentioned that the color of opium resembles thick oxgall, and this equally bitter vegetable product could have been given the name gall by the people. There can be no doubt that the ancient Israelites knew of the sleep-inducing poppy, belonging to the family of *Papaveraceae*, since it is native to the lands of the east. The ancient Egyptians knew about unripe poppy capsules and how to extract the milky sap which, when dried, became opium. This sap contains the now commonly known opium alkaloids (for example, morphine and codeine) which play a major role in modern

---

[13] The word "gall" is found in the King James text.

medicine. The Greeks also knew about opium long before the birth of Christ. Theophrastus, a pupil of Aristotle, explained the method of obtaining the sap by incising the capsules and described its medical application. The rich oil obtained from the poppy seeds was used in ancient times to alleviate tumors. It contains alkaloids which are not too poisonous. Poppy seed is also used as a culinary oil and in the manufacture of paint.

Lemon Peel

It is not known for sure whether the fruit from the *Citrus Limonum Risso* or *Citrius medica L.,* of the family of *Rutaceae,* was known in the time of Moses. It is, however, almost certain that lemons were in use by the Israelites by 100 B.C.

> Howbeit on the fifteenth day of the seventh month, when ye have gathered in the fruits of the land, ye shall keep the feast of the Lord seven days; on the first day shall be a solemn rest, and on the eighth day shall be a solemn rest. And ye shall take you on the first day the fruit of goodly trees, branches of palm-trees, and boughs of thick trees, and willows of the brook, and ye shall rejoice before the Lord your God seven days.
> (Leviticus 23:39, 40)

During the harvest festivities, Israelites used to carry fruits called *ethrogiem,* which were a kind of orange-apple. According to some Hebrew rabbis, "the fruit of goodly trees" means lemons.

Alexander the Great, in a fit of tyranny, so angered the Israelites during the Feast of the Tabernacles that they hurled lemons at him in their rage. Carrying one of these fruits is a symbol of all the good things which God has given.

The approximately 10-14 meter high lemon tree is native to Persia and Medea and must have been taken from there to the Mediterranean region, where it is now cultivated in abundance. The essential lemon oil, used medicinally as a taste corrigent, can be obtained by squeezing fresh lemon peel.

Raisins and Currants

The most noble plant on earth, the grapevine, is one of the gifts with which the Lord favors the land of his chosen people. The juice obtained by squeezing the fruit of the vine was such a common drink in Israel that it was considered one of man's primary necessities of life. Fermented grape juice was an everyday drink. Just as today, wine was famed for its stimulating influence and censured for its misuse. Taken in suitable quantities, it has remained to this day an important medicine.

After leaving the Ark, Noah tilled the ground and planted a vineyard (Genesis 9:20); it was he who discovered the pleasures of wine and the misery of immoderate use—he became drunk and stripped himself naked with the well-known consequence that Canaan was cursed by his father as a punishment for his curiosity. (Genesis 9:25) We can, however, establish that the injurious effect of wine is usually of a passing nature, since Noah lived another three hundred and fifty years.

It is not surprising to find that wine is not forgotten in biblical poetry, when the bride in The Song of Songs says to the bridegroom, as an image of caressing:

>... I would cause thee to drink of spiced wine,
>Of the juice of my pomegranate.
>
>(The Song of Songs 8:2)

The importance attached to a good wine harvest is evident in Deuteronomy where, among the laws concerning the waging of war, several people are given the freedom to return home, including anyone who has planted a vineyard but has not yet made use of it: "... let him go and return unto his house, lest he die in the battle . . ." (Deuteronomy 20:6)

It is clear from the lamentation about Moab that the wine harvest was a time for great happiness:

> And gladness and joy are taken away
> Out of the fruitful field;
> And in the vineyards there shall be no singing,
> Neither shall there be shouting;
> No treader shall tread out wine in the presses;
> I have made the vintage shout to cease.
> (Isaiah 16:10)

The whole of Israel was called the vineyard of the Lord, who tended it as a careful farmer would tend his vineyard. The vineyard had to be enclosed in order to protect it from wild animals; the vats were hewed out of the mountain and a tower was added that functioned as a watch house. (Isaiah 5:2)

Vitis vinifera, of the family of *Vitaceae,* was the plant mentioned in early times and is, along with many different types and varieties of slender, climbing plants, still the supplier of wine. Raisins and currants are the dried fruits of different varieties of grape. In antiquity, as today, they were used to prepare delicious kinds of bread. The Egyptian who showed David which road the Amalekites had taken was first given bread and then raisins to bring him back to health:

> And they gave him a piece of a cake of figs, and two clusters of raisins; and when he had eaten, his spirit came back to him; for he had eaten no bread, nor drunk any water, three days and three nights.
> (I Samuel 30:12)

The ancient Hebrews prepared vinegar from wine and other kinds of alcoholic drinks, such as the so-called *sicera* (beers).[14] The ancient Israelites made a distinction between wine and beer vinegar, neither of which could be taken by a Nazirite (i.e. an initiate, a recluse):

And the Lord spoke unto Moses, saying: Speak unto the children of Israel, and say unto them: When either man or woman shall clearly utter a vow, the vow of a Nazirite, to consecrate himself unto the Lord, he shall abstain from wine and strong drink: he shall drink no vinegar of wine, or vinegar of strong drink, neither shall he drink any liquor of grapes . . .

(Numbers 6:1-3)

Vinegar was used, either alone or mixed with oil or water, as an astringent for the treatment of toothache or in the form of compresses for bleeding and rheumatic lumbago. The word "vinegar" is a combination of *vin* (wine) and *aigre* (sour), a liquid which must have been concentrated wine vinegar that would certainly have offered no refreshment, and indeed was even mentioned in the Bible in the same breath as poisoned food:

"They put poison in my food and gave me vinegar when I was thirsty."

(Psalms 69:22)

It is not possible to state with certainty whether vinegar should also be taken to be a narcotic, as this is the same combination as was given to Jesus immediately before the crucifixion: ". . . and there he was offered a draught of wine mixed with gall; but when he had tasted it he would not drink." (Matthew 27:34)

Other translations of the Bible give the word "vinegar" in this context. The vinegar that Jesus drank just before he gave

---

[14]Sicera includes drinks made by the process of fermentation (from dates, for example).

up the ghost would have been the drink prepared from sour wine. (Matthew 27:48)

Reference to the bad effect of vinegar on men's teeth and the caustic action on skin can be found in Proverbs:

> As vinegar to the teeth, and as smoke to the eyes,
> So is the sluggard to them that send him.
> (Proverbs 10:26)

> As one that taketh off a garment in cold weather, and as vinegar upon nitre,
> So is he that singeth songs to a heavy heart.
> (Proverbs 25:20)

Vinegar is also mentioned in Ruth, but this probably means wine vinegar served for refreshment since Boaz gave it to Ruth as a reward for her love for her mother-in-law, a blood relation of Boaz: "And Boaz said unto her at meal-time: 'Come hither, and eat of the bread, and dip thy morsel in the vinegar." (Ruth 2:14)

Pistachio Nuts

This is an oblong nut from *Pistacia vera* which is commonly confused with *Pistacia terebinthus* (see Turpentine, page 91). Both are members of the *Anacardiaceae* family. *Pistacia vera* grows in Palestine, Syria and Persia, but not in Egypt, a fact which led to Jacob's recommending his sons to include these nuts as a gift for Joseph when they took Benjamin to Egypt:

> Their father Israel said to them, 'If it must be so, then do this: take in your baggage, as a gift for the man, some of the produce for which our country is

famous: a little balsam, a little honey, gum tragacanth, myrrh, pistachio nuts, and almonds. (Genesis 43:11)[15]

Coriander Fruits

Coriandrum sativum, belonging to the family of *Umbelliferae,* has double podded fruits, yellow-brown on the outside. This pale brown color resembles that of fresh manna. Where the Bible refers to seed, it in fact probably also means the fruit. The word "seed" is often used to describe fruit when the latter is small. Thus one speaks of aniseed, caraway seed, fennel seed, etc. when referring to the fruits of these herbs belonging to the family of *Umbelliferae,* since the whole fruit is sown in the ground.

> And the house of Israel called the name thereof Manna; and it was like coriander seed, white; and the taste of it was like wafers made with honey.
> (Exodus 16:31)

Coriander is grown throughout Europe; the fruit, with its special aromatic fragrance, is used medicinally as a taste corrigent.

Cummin Fruit

These fruits are well known from their use in cheese. They come from *Cuminum cyminum,* an umbelliferous plant, native to Egypt and extensively grown in southern Europe.

---

[15]This translation is from the New English version of the Bible. Other translations do not name specific variety of "nuts."

Cummin is mentioned with mint and dill in the Gospel according to St. Matthew (23:23). (See Peppermint Leaves, page 51.) Cummin was used by the ancient Israelites as a healing remedy following circumcision.

It is stated in Isaiah that the Lord regulates everything, even the treatment of agricultural produce:

> When he hath made plain the face thereof,
> Doth he not cast abroad the black cummin, and scatter the cummin,
> And put in the wheat in rows and the barley in the appointed place
> And the spelt in the border thereof?
> For He doth instruct him aright;
> His God doth teach him.
> For the black cummin is not threshed with a threshing-sledge,
> Neither is a cart-wheel turned about upon the cummin;
> But the black cummin is beaten out with a staff,
> And the cummin with a rod.
> (Isaiah 28:25-27)

Dill Fruit

A member of the *Umbelliferae,* whose fruit is much sought after for seasoning, because of the aromatic, essential oil it contains, is dill, *Anethum graveolens.* Dill grows wild in Palestine. When it was cultivated, a tenth had to be handed over to the priests. Dill is also mentioned in the passage quoted under Peppermint Leaves from Matthew (23:23). Dill is used as a stomachic in folk medicine.

Mulberries

The mulberry tree originally came from Persia and Asia Minor. It is the drupe of *Morus nigra* which provides *sirupus mororum,* a taste corrigent for medicines. *Morus alba* can also be found in Palestine. Silk worms prefer to eat the leaves of this variety. The mulberry tree, from the family of *Moraceae,* only grows in the lower regions of Palestine and was evidently also cultivated there since Amos denies being a prophet but is simply: "... a herdsman, and a dresser of sycomore-trees ..." (Amos 7:14)

The "sycomore" or "sycamine" is the black mulberry tree (Hebrew *shiqmah*). The fact that mulberry trees were common is echoed in Kings:

> And the king made silver to be in Jerusalem as stones, and cedars made he to be as the sycomore-trees that are in the Lowland, for abundance.
> (I Kings 10:27)

The very light, durable wood from the gnarly trunk was also used for a variety of purposes.

Figs

The fig, still a popular fruit, appeared on the table in antiquity in homes of rich and poor alike and was a delicious, important food. The sighs heaved by the Israelites when they were in the desert of Zin, led there by Aaron and Moses, were for the fig, mentioned in the same breath as water:

> And wherefore have ye made us to come up out of Egypt, to bring us in unto this evil place? it is no place of seed, or of figs, or of vines, or of

pomegranates; neither is there any water to drink."
(Numbers 20:5)

It is also referred to in the poetry of the ancient Hebrews:

> The fig-tree putteth forth her green figs,
> And the vines in blossom give forth their fragrance.
> Arise, my love, my fair one, and come away.
> (The Song of Songs 2:13)

This is not surprising as not only was the fruit of the fig tree popular, but the shade offered by its wide-spread branches with large leaves was much sought after too. Living under the shade and eating the fruit of one's own fig tree was part of the imperturbable, homely peace enjoyed by the Israelites under their wise King Solomon: "... And Judah and Israel dwelt safely, every man under his vine and under his fig-tree, from Dan even to Beer-sheba ..." (I Kings 5:5)[16] The fig tree is also one of the first trees mentioned in the Bible. After the fall of man, Adam and Eve stitched fig leaves together and made themselves loincloths. (Genesis 3:7)

In ancient times figs had a medicinal use as an external remedy. They were pounded to a kind of pulp, as we do today with linseed meal, and applied to inflammation and ulceration. The prophet Isaiah advises the devout King Hezekiah to apply a cake of figs on a malignant swelling from which he would die; Hezekiah lived another fifteen years. (II Kings 20:7)

Today, syrup of figs is made and used as a laxative. This hollow, fleshy, common receptacle, with its large number of stone fruits (seeds), from *Ficus carica* of the *Moraceae* family, is now popularly used as an internal remedy. The fig tree is cultivated in the areas around the Mediterranean.

---

[16]This verse is I Kings 4:25 in the King James version of the Bible.

Apples and Quinces

The Hebrew name *thapuah* ("that which smells [sweet]") for an apple tree, refers to the pleasant smell of the fruit. In The Song of Songs, the enraptured lover says of his loved one:

> ... And the smell of thy countenance like
> apples...
> (The Song of Songs 7:9)

Since the apple tree is seldom found in hot countries and usually fails to flourish there, it has been suggested that the tree mentioned in several passages in the Bible could be the quince, which also belongs to the family of *Rosaceae* and even now can be found more abundantly in the Holy Land than the apple. But this suggestion is unnecessary since the finer varieties of apples and pears came to us from Asia Minor and Syria, and apple trees grow today not only on the higher lying regions of the Sinai but also on the tablelands of Hebron and lower lying regions.

Although the extract or tincture of apples and quinces have more or less the same medicinal significance, the apple has more value in daily use than the quince since the latter's acid taste prevents it from being a popular consumer item. It is probable that the apple tree indicated in the Bible is the *Pyrus malus;* this would better explain the praise sung of its fruit:

> As an apple-tree among the trees of the wood,
> So is my beloved among the sons.
> Under its shadow I delighted to sit,
> And its fruit was sweet to my taste.
> (The Song of Songs 2:3)

Colocynth Apples

The fruits of *Citrullus colocynthis* have acquired a certain renown in the Bible: when eaten as "wild gourds," they at first appeared to be inedible, but following Elisha's miracle, they could indeed be eaten.

> And Elisha came again to Gilgal; and there was a dearth in the land; and the sons of the prophets were sitting before him; and he said unto his servant: 'Set on the great pot, and see the pottage for the sons of the prophets.' And one went out into the field to gather herbs, and found a wild vine, and gathered thereof wild gourds his lap full, and came and shred them into the pot of pottage; for they knew them not. So they poured out for the men to eat. And it came to pass, as they were eating of the pottage, that they cried out, and said: 'O man of God, there is death in the pot.' And they could not eat thereof. But he said: 'Then bring meal.' And he cast it into the pot; and he said: 'Pour out for the people, that they may eat.' And there was no harm in the pot.
> (II Kings 4:38-41)

Other translations of the Bible refer to "wild cucumbers." This is conceivable since the colocynth belongs to the same family *(Cucurbitaceae)* as the cuccumis which provides gherkins; this would relate the colocynth to twining, climbing, herbaceous plants. The colocynth fruit is an attractive yellow, apple-shaped cucumber fruit and even served as a decorative motif for the temple. "And the cedar on the house within was carved with knops [or gourds] and open flowers. . ." (I Kings 6:18)

Knops or gourds are colocynth apples. It was evidently the very bitter taste of these fruits that alarmed the sons of the prophets and caused men to cry out "There is death in the pot." It is not absolutely clear if Elisha really added "meal" to these bitter apples, thereby simply improving the taste, or if he added something else which made the bitter glucoside colocynthine lose its taste.

The colocynth is used now, as in early medical practice, as a purgative. Their native lands are Persia and Arabia;

colocynths also come from Spain where they are widely cultivated.

Cucumbers

During their flight through the desert, the Israelites lamented the lack of cucumbers, which were available in abundance in the land of Egypt (see Garlic, page 25). The ancient Hebrews cultivated this fruit after their safe arrival in Canaan. However, the Lord reproached ungrateful Israel for its ungodliness. The land is truly wretched:

> And the daughter of Zion is left
> As a booth in a vineyard,
> As a lodge in a garden of cucumbers,
> As a besieged city.
> (Isaiah 1:8)

The cucumber plant *Cucumis sativus* belongs to the family of *Cucurbitaceae* that grows with tendrils, and was abundantly cultivated in ancient Israel. Watch was kept over them, as in the case of grapes, since cucumbers were an important food. This plant has no great medicinal significance. Like melon, cucumber was used in Palestine as a refreshing food for feverish patients.

Melons

Also members of the *Cucurbitaceae* family, like the cucumber, *Cucumis melo* and the watermelon *Cucumis citrullus,* have the same medicinal significance as the cucumber above. Melons were a very popular food, held in high esteem by Israelite exiles in Egypt (see Garlic, page 25). On their trek through the dry sand, the wanderer particularly yearned for watermelon, which contains refreshing liquid.

Mustard Seed

One of the parables of Jesus goes as follows:

> '... The kingdom of Heaven is like a mustard-seed, which a man took and sowed in his field. As a seed, mustard is smaller than any other; but when it has grown it is bigger than any garden-plant; it becomes a tree, big enough for the birds to come and roost among its branches.'
> (Matthew 13:31, 32)

It is also evident from Matthew that the seed of the mustard plant was considered to be very small in relation to that of other cultivated plants:

> He answered, 'Your faith is too small. I tell you this: if you have faith no bigger even than a mustard-seed, you will say to this mountain, "Move from here to there!", and it will move; nothing will prove impossible for you.'
> (Matthew 17:20)

Both *Brassica nigra* (black mustard) and *Brassica alba* (white mustard) belong to the family of *Cruciferae,* produce small seeds and are cultivated in Europe. Although the plant does not resemble a tree, it apparently grows very large in a hot climate. With respect to the fact that Jesus refers to a "tree" in which the birds of the heaven can nest, there is no reason to suppose that our own well-known mustard plant is not indicated. It cannot be stated with any certainty to which country the mustard plant is native, since this plant has been cultivated everywhere since time immemorial and is abundantly found in the wild, however, there are some grounds for suggesting that these plants originally came from the southeastern Mediterranean region. Mustard was used in ancient times both as seasoning and as a medicinal remedy. Mustard in the form of a mustard plaster and mustard paper, is intended to have an irritating and pain relieving effect on rheumatism. The glucoside sinigrin reacts in the presence of water to form essential oil of mustard, bringing about the stimulating taste and smell.

Linseed

Flax is one of the oldest known cultivated plants, *Linum usitasissimum,* belonging to the family of *Linaceae,* and was already being grown in Egypt in 1400 B.C. Ancient Egyptian wall paintings show the whole process of working flax, and mummies from that period were wrapped in linen.

The word "linen" brings to mind the image of a busy housewife. In the Bible, the preparation of flax is recorded as one of her virtues:

> She seeketh wool and flax,
> And worketh willingly with her hands.
> (Proverbs 31:13)

After the blooming period, the flax is pulled out, tied in bundles and placed in water so as to partially rot; this process makes it easier to separate the fibers from the stems. The ancient Israelites dried the flax by laying it on the roofs of their houses; because of this, Rahab was able to hide the spies sent by Joshua to Jericho who were sought by the king of Jericho: "But she had brought them up to the roof, and hid them with the stalks of flax, which she had spread out upon the roof." (Joshua 2:6)

Linseed meal was used by the ancient Hebrews for poultices, and Theophrastus referred to the action of linseed slime for medicinal purposes. This is still used today for the treatment of inflammation of the urinary organs. Oil extracted from linseed has both technical and medicinal applications. When mixed with lime water, it is a well-known remedy for burns.

Ricinus Seed

The castor-oil plant (*Ricinus communis*) is also known as Miracle Tree, and probably got this name because of its extraordinarily rapid growth. In a warm climate, it can grow to a height of forty feet in a few months. However, just as rapidly as it grows, it can also die if the leaves are damaged by caterpillars. The castor-oil plant is a tropical African and Asiatic herb, naturalized in all tropical countries. Castor oil is extracted from the ricinus seed by cold press methods and is used as a lubricant in soap and as a cathartic. The medicinal properties of castor oil must have been known in biblical times; we can see reference to the tree itself in Jonah:

> Then the Lord God ordained that a climbing gourd (a castor-oil plant) should grow up over his head to throw its shade over him and relieve his distress, and Jonah was grateful for the gourd. But at dawn the next day God ordained that a worm should attack the gourd, and it withered; and at sunrise God ordained that a scorching wind should blow up from the east.
> (Jonah 4:6-8)[17]

Milk Thistle Seed

The seed of *Carduus marianus,* belonging to the *Compositae* family, is used as a folk remedy for jaundice. The marian thistle is native to the Mediterranean region and is also found in European vegetable gardens as a weed, blooming with purple flowers. This plant is one of the thistles mentioned many times in the Bible. (See also Greater Celandine Herb, page 45.)

Almonds

The almond tree found in Asia and Africa is abundantly cultivated in the lands around the Mediterranean in two

---

[17]From the *New English Bible.*

varieties: *Amygdalus dulcis,* the sweet almond, and *Amygdalus amarus,* the bitter almond tree. Both types of almond contain a rich, fluid oil with a pleasant taste. Bitter almonds also contain a glucoside, amygdalin, which in the presence of water is split by the enzyme emulsin, into benzaldehyde, a sugar, and the highly poisonous prussic acid. The hard exterior of European almonds is the inside of the fruit wall; the seed with its thin, brown seed coat and white seed lobes lies within.

In Genesis, Jacob peels strips of bark from fresh branches of willow, almond and plane and lays them in the water troughs for the rutting goats. (Genesis 30:37) The Hebrew name for *Prunus amygdalus* is "the one who is awake," perhaps because it blooms before all other fruit trees with pale pink flowers. Jeremiah uses it, in a play on words, to indicate that the Lord is "awake" and no delay in the threatened punishment can cause doubts as to the certainty of the judgment of God:

> Moreover the word of the Lord came unto me, saying: 'Jeremiah, what seest thou?' And I said: 'I see a rod of an almond-tree.' Then said the Lord unto me: 'Thou hast well seen; for I watch over My word to perform it.'
> (Jeremiah 1:11, 12)

It is not surprising that the almond tree has such beautiful blossoms when one considers the fact that it is a member of the *Rosaceae* family.

FIBERS AND AMORPHOUS RAW MATERIALS

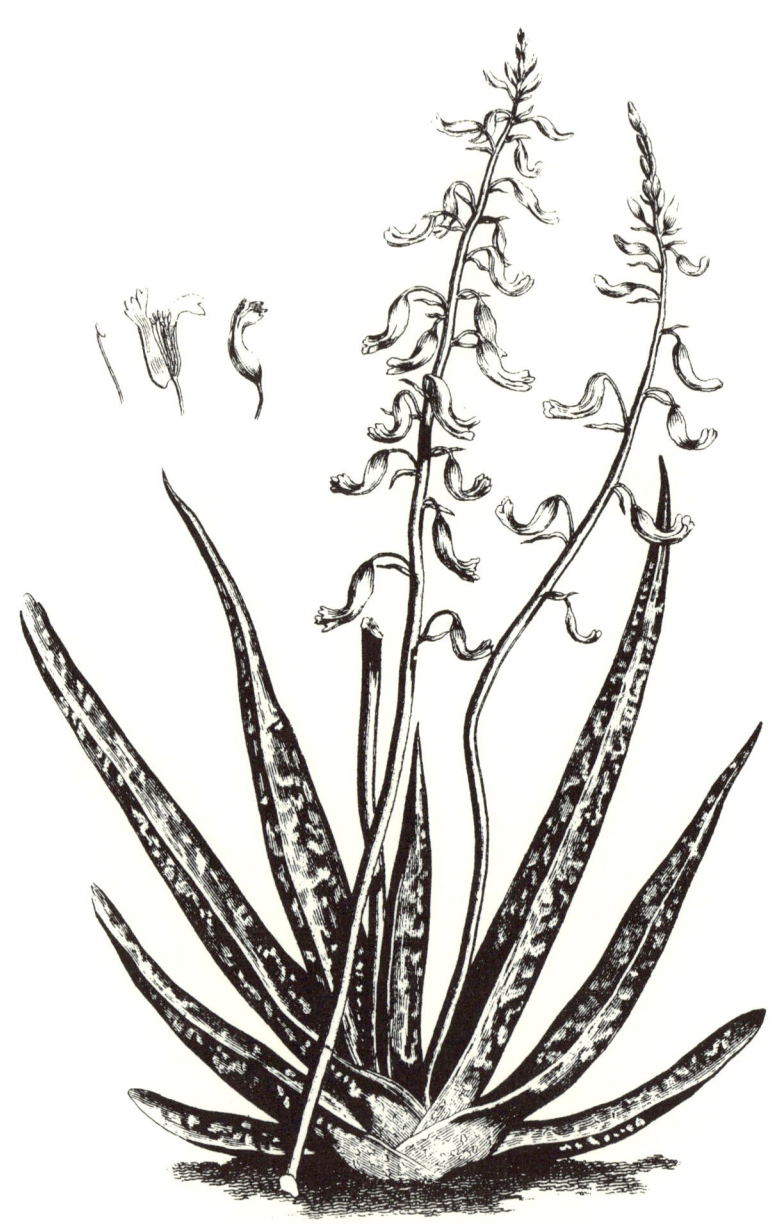

Aloe

Cotton

When the seed box of different types of *Gossypium* bursts open, the seeds appear with the surrounding cotton in the form of a ball. This cotton consists of fibers which appear on the seeds. (See Gossypium Bark, page 37.)

Gallnuts

Gallnuts, or oak apples, are abnormal growths caused by the sting of a gallfly on the branches of different varieties of oak. (See Oak Bark, page 35.)

Manna

The tamarisk, a sacred tree, is described as an evergreen with fine, wide-spread branches and beautiful pink blossoms. According to De Visser, it sweats a sugary kind of fluid which could be manna. The manna which the children of Israel ate for forty years during their trek through the desert until they reached the inhabited land of Canaan is probably the same food of the desert which can be found today on the Sinai Peninsula, and which the Arabs smear on their bread. The tamarisk *(el-Tarfah)* is most likely the *Tamarix mannifera,* a shrub belonging to the family of *Tamaricaceae,* commonly found in the watery regions in the neighborhood of the Sinai mountains. "And Abraham planted a tamarisk-tree in Beer-sheba, and called there on the name of the Lord, the Everlasting God." (Genesis 21:33)

A light brown sap, which thickens as it dries, drips from the twigs of this shrub: "... it was like coriander seed, white..." (Exodus 16:31) This probably means light brown, like the color of coriander seed. Manna is compared with honey, but is far from being so pleasant to European taste. The Bedouins call manna a "gift from heaven" and say that it "rains down from heaven." In Numbers it is stated how manna was used:

> Now the manna was like coriander seed, and the appearance thereof as the appearance of bdellium [a transparent, wax-like resin]. The people went about, and gathered it, and ground it in mills, or beat it in mortars, and seethed it in pots, and made cakes of it; and the taste of it was as the taste of a cake baked with oil. And when the dew fell upon the camp in the night, the manna fell upon it.
> (Numbers 11:7-9)

The manna of the Bible is not the same as that used in pharmacy, which comes from *Fraxinus ornus,* a plant from the *Oleaceae* family, and which is also a low tree with pink blossoms. Pharmaceutical manna, which contains 80-90% mannite or mannatol (this is in fact 6 carbon atom alcohol) and other different types of sugar, has an important nutritional value. This manna is exclusively collected on the north coast of Sicily by making horizontal incisions in the bark of the manna tree, which exude a brown-blue fluorescent, bitter tasting liquid that turns white and crystalline after a few hours and soon after loses its bitter taste.

Wheat

Wheat was already cultivated far back in earliest times. Wheat flour was not only used to bake bread but was also utilized as a medicinal remedy. It was chewed raw and placed on ulcers which would then soon come to a head and burst. The starch from the grain was used by the ancient Hebrews as a powder in all kinds of skin remedies; it is still used today for the same purpose and can also still be found on the dressing table.

The plant *Triticum vulgare* is a *Graminae* which is now a principal supplier of food for the whole world. In the Bible, the wheat harvest is referred to in the first Book of Moses (Genesis 30:14). As proof of his love for his sons, the Lord will take them to the land of Canaan: "... a good land ... a land of wheat and barley ..." (Deuteronomy 8:7, 8)

Tragacanth

De Visser states that Tragacanth was one of the gifts which Jacob gave to his sons to offer to Joseph (Genesis 43:11). Although the English authorized version refers to "spicery and myrrh," other translations refer to "gum and myrrh." This "gum" could have been tragacanth, as tragacanth is indeed a kind of gum. Different types of *Astralagus,* from the family of *Papilionaceae,* exude a thick fluid when the trunk is incised; this fluid rapidly dries into white, sickle-shaped strips, with wavy stripes and an insipid taste. Tragacanth consists of pith cells which have changed into gum. The types of *Astralagus* mentioned are generally low shrubs which grow on the mountain slopes of Asia Minor and Persia.

Olibanum

This highly regarded gum resin is frequently mentioned at the same time as myrrh in the Bible. In order to obtain this gum resin, incisions are made in the trunks of trees belonging to the *Boswellia* group, for example *Boswellia carterii*. The resin runs out and dries on contact with air into grains that are either oblong or more spherical with a 1-2½ cm. diameter. The grains are brittle, pale yellow and dull. When heated they partially melt and exude an intoxicating but very pleasant smell. According to the laws given to Moses by the Lord, a separate altar had to be used for the burning of holy incense:

> And thou shalt make an altar to burn incense upon; of acacia-wood shalt thou make it.... And thou shalt overlay it with pure gold ...
>
> (Exodus 30:1, 3)

Incense was also added to the offering of bread:

> And thou shalt take fine flour, and bake twelve cakes thereof: two tenth parts of an ephah shall be in one cake. And thou shalt set them in two rows, six in a row, upon the pure table before the Lord. And thou shalt put pure frankincense with each row, that it may be to the bread for a memorial-part, even an offering made by fire unto the Lord.
>
> (Leviticus 24:5-7)

The trees which supplied incense appear to have flourished particularly well in Egypt. In Isaiah it is believed that the inhabitants of Sheba, a land to the south of Ethiopia, will come to Jerusalem when the light of the Lord's glory rises over Israel.

> ...All coming from Sheba;
> They shall bring gold and frankincense,
> And shall proclaim the praises of the Lord.
>
> (Isaiah 60:6)

Boswellia carterii, from the family of *Burseraceae,* is a tree which is now commonly found in Arabia and east Africa.

Myrrh

Myrrh flows naturally from the trunks and branches of a small tree, *Commiphora abyssinica,* belonging to the family of *Burseraceae,* native to southern Arabia and northeastern Africa. Pale yellow, oil-like myrrh drips from the dull gray bark, and after drying forms irregularly shaped or round light or dark brown grains that have a whitish tinge here and there. Dried myrrh is hard and brittle, tastes bitter and has an aromatic scent due to its constituents: volatile oil, resin and a bitter substance. In the very earliest days of Israel, myrrh was considered to be an important ingredient, and the Lord charges Moses to use it for the holy anointing oil. Myrrh was also used for perfume. It surrounds Solomon's litter and is observed by the daughters of Jerusalem.

> Who is this that cometh up out of the wilderness
> Like pillars of smoke,
> Perfumed with myrrh and frankincense . . .
> (The Song of Songs 3.6)

Myrrh was also highly favored as a toilet article. The maidens who were led before King Ahasuerus, who would choose a new queen from among them, were purified for twelve months, according to the law for women: six months with oil of myrrh and six with balsams and other means of beautification. (Esther 2:12) Myrrh was also used for burial of the dead:

> He was joined by Nicodemus (the man who had first visited Jesus by night), who brought with him a mixture of myrrh and aloes, more than half a hundredweight. They took the body of Jesus and wrapped it, with the spices, in strips of linen cloth according to Jewish burial-customs.
> (John 19:39, 40)

St. Mark states that a drink of myrrh was given to Jesus and was refused by him: "And they gave him to drink wine mingled with myrrh: but he received it not."(Mark 15:23)[18] St. Matthew says that they gave him "wine mingled with gall." (27:34) (See Poppy Capsules, page 62.)

Myrrh is still used as a local anesthetic: myrrh and scurvy grass is a well-known folk remedy for toothache. Tincture of myrrh is also used for this purpose.

Bdellium

Havilah was a country southeast of the Dead Sea in the Arabian desert. Here one could find the gum resin "bdellium" which, like myrrh, consists of gum, resin and essential oil, and was used to replace the latter. The smell of bdellium is less pleasant than that of myrrh and the color is more greenish-black. It comes from a plant called *Commiphora africana* which, like the myrrh plant, belongs to the family of *Burseraceae*.

> And a river went out of Eden to water the garden; and from thence it was parted, and became four heads. The name of the first is Pishon; that is it which compasseth the whole land of Havilah, where there is gold; and the gold of that land is good; there is bdellium and the onyx stone.
> (Genesis 2:10-12)

Galbanum

One cannot say with certainty for what purpose the gum resin "galbanum" was added to the holy perfume. The smell

---

[18]This translation is from the King James version of the Bible. The New English version describes this mixture as "drugged wine."

is indeed aromatic but not pleasant when burned. It is possible that the smoke of galbanum was attributed with beneficial action and for this reason received a place of honor. (Exodus 30:35) Galbanum was also used internally, but is today generally used externally in the form of plasters.

In addition to the resin that is naturally exuded, resin is also produced and collected by cutting away the stems above the roots. *Ferula galbaniflua* is a herbaceous plant, approximately two meters high, belonging to the *Umbelliferae,* and is commonly found on the Persian tablelands. Galbanum appears in the form of sticky brown grains which usually cling together.

Resin

Colophonium, the resin from various types of *Pinus,* belonging to the family of *Coniferae,* was undoubtedly known to the ancient Hebrews, since the "fir-tree" is repeatedly mentioned in the Scriptures. According to the prophet, the light of the Lord shall rise over Israel and all nations will have to yield the wealth of their land or be punished by destruction.

> For the nation and kingdom that will not serve thee shall perish; yea, those nations shall be utterly wasted. The glory of Leb-a-non shall come unto thee, the fir tree,[19] the pine tree, and the box together, to beautify the place of my sanctuary; and I will make the place of my feet glorious.
> (Isaiah 60:12, 13)

Musical instruments evidently were manufactured from fir wood. When David goes with the people to fetch the ark

---

[19]This translation comes from the King James Version of the Bible. Other versions cite this tree as "cypress." The two terms, in this context, are interchangeable.

from Baale Judah, after conquering the Philistines, they go before the ark.

> And David and all the house of Israel played before the Lord on all manner of instruments made of fir wood, even on harps, and on psalteries, and on timbrels, and on cornets, and on cymbals.[20]
>
> (II Samuel 6:5)

It is highly probable that the name colophonium has its origin in the city of Colophon on the coast of Asia Minor, since the area surrounding this place formerly supplied quantities of pine tree resin, known as "resin from Colophonia." Colophonium is frequently utilized medicinally for making plasters. The resin was also used for this purpose in the ancient lands of the east. The principal supplier of resin has always been *Pinus silvestris* which grows in Asia and Europe. This supplies turpentine which runs out of the trunk in the form of balsam. When turpentine oil has been distilled from this, colophonium remains in the form of brittle, transparent pieces, light brown in color. This substance has technical uses in the manufacture of varnishes, paints and for treating violin strings.[21]

Mastic

This resin comes from the trunk and branches of *Pistacia Lentiscus,* a shrub from the family of *Anacardiaceae,* native to the Greek archipelago. Its name is of Greek origin; *mastichare* is to chew, and mastic was chewed for the purpose of sweetening the breath. In Hebrew, this resin was called *zori,* which can be translated as "balsam." When

---
[20]From the King James version of the Bible.
[21]The tree that supplies turpentine is not the terebinth or turpentine tree of the Bible. (See Turpentine in this section.)

Joseph's brothers sat down to a meal after throwing him in the pit,

> ... they lifted up their eyes and looked, and, behold, a caravan of Ishmaelites came from Gilead, with their camels bearing spicery and balm and ladanum, going to carry it down to Egypt.
> (Genesis 37:25)

A footnote in one version of the Bible gives an alternative translation for "balm" as "mastic." The word balm in Ezekiel is given where mastic could equally well be indicated. It is the last of the six products which were brought to the Tyrian market from Israel:

> Judah, and the land of Israel, they were thy traffickers; they traded for thy merchandise wheat of Minnith, and balsam, and honey, and oil, and balm.
> (Ezekiel 27:17)

Mastic is exuded naturally and from incisions in the form of a thick fluid mass and dries on contact with the air into round or tear-shaped grains. These are pale yellow and more or less transparent. It turns soft and sticky in the mouth, and when burned emanates an aromatic perfume. Mastic was used medicinally in ancient times: internally for the treatment of intestinal complaints and venereal disease; externally in cases of rheumatism. It now has technical applications in the form of glue and varnish, and in perfumery items.

Labdanum

De Visser suggests that labdanum or ladanum is referred to in the Hebrew text where the King James version of the Bible speaks of myrrh: "... with their camels bearing spicery and balm and myrrh ..." (Genesis 37:25) This resin is exuded especially during the summer period from the green hairy branches and lanceolate leaves of *Cistus creticus,* a shrub from the family of *Cistaceae.* It is principally gathered today in Crete by monks: they rub their belts against it and then harvest what adheres. In Israel the resin was collected by driving goats alongside the shrubs so that the sticky substance clung to their hair. Labdanum is a dark brown tough substance with a smell similar to that of balsamandis, and is often used as a substitute for styrax. The word ladanum formerly indicated a mixture of incense, sand and labdanum thinly rolled into sticks that were then twisted spirally around each other and burned. While labdanum is principally used in perfumery, it was and still is used to soften ulcers.

Turpentine

De Visser describes the terebinth, or turpentine, tree as having a strong trunk, brown bark, thin branches, a regularly shaped crown and oval lanceolate leaves, which are first red, then dark green. According to Zeller, the terebinth tree has a widely branched, irregular crown, with branches that have a strong tendency to droop downwards (particularly in the male tree). This corresponds with the description of the death of Absalom:

> And Absalom chanced to meet the servants of David. And Absalom was riding upon his mule, and the mule went under the thick boughs of a great terebinth, and his head caught hold of the terebinth, and he was taken up between the heaven and the earth; and the mule that was under him went on.
> (II Samuel 18:9)
> ...And he took three darts in his hand, and thrust them through the heart of Absalom, while he was yet alive in the midst of the terebinth. And ten

young men that bore Joab's armour compassed
about and smote Absalom, and slew him.
(II Samuel 18:14, 15)

Incisions in the trunk and branches of the terebinth produce resin: it is a turpentine that has a pleasant smell and taste. This turpentine tree, which particularly flourishes in southern Palestine and which is one of the few trees on the tableland of Ammon, Moab and Hesbon, is probably *Pistacia terebinthus.* What we know as turpentine comes principally from different types of *Pinus* (see Resin in this chapter). The taste of our turpentine is not pleasant and the leaves of the biblical turpentine are not needle-shaped; those of the *Coniferae,* to which *Pinus* belongs, are. *Pistacia terebinthus* belongs to the *Anacardiaceae,* a family which grows extensively in hot climates. The plants belonging to this group usually have one-seeded fruits that are generally edible; this corresponds to the statement that the terebinth has small nuts with an edible kernel. These are probably not pistachio nuts which come from *Pistacia vera,* related, like the terebinth, to *Pistacia Lentiscus,* which provides mastic. (See Pistachio Nuts, page 67 and Mastic, page 88.)

Cedar Oil

Apart from its use as an alternative to sandalwood oil, cedar oil is used for microscopic purposes. The somewhat yellow essential oil is principally obtained from cedar-wood chip waste matter left over from the manufacture of pencils. The cedar oil which is used medicinally generally comes from *Juniperis virginiana,* a conifer which grows in America. Also available commercially is cedar oil from *Cedrus Libani,* likewise a conifer, which, as the name indicates, comes from eastern Asia. Since cedar does not grow in the desert, there is a clear case of invention in Leviticus 14:6 where the priest asks for cedar wood to be brought for use in the purification of lepers. (See Hyssop Herb, page 47.) Since the ancient

Hebrews attached great value to the disinfectant action of essential oils, it would not be improbable for cedar wood to have played a more significant part in this ceremony than is apparent in the Bible. If we think of the "living water" used here as "boiling water" into which the cedar wood was thrown, we approach the process by which essential oil is obtained from cedar wood today. This takes place through distillation by steam of powdered or finely chopped cedar wood. Cedar from Lebanon would undoubtedly have emanated a very strong smell and today the oil is introduced into water for the same purpose: to be inhaled in cases of bronchitis. The authors of Leviticus also possibly expected the vapor, impregnated with aromatic cedar oil, to have a disinfectant action on the skin of the leper. I can however find no confirmation for my supposition.

Lebanese cedar is referred to by name when Solomon requests Hirom, the King of Tyre, to send his servants to come and cut down these trees for the construction of the Temple:

> 'Now therefore command thou that they hew me cedar-trees out of Lebanon; and my servants shall be with thy servants; and I will give thee hire for thy servants according to all that thou shalt say; for thou knowest that there is not among us any that hath skill to hew timber like unto the Zidonians.'
>
> (I Kings 5:20)

Styrax

"Stacte" is mentioned on page 9 as one of the ingredients of the holy perfume. This would have been "styrax" from *Styrax officinalis.* The styrax that is currently used medicinally is a sticky, grayish-brown balsam, and comes from the wood of *Liquidambar orientalis,* a tree resembling a plane tree from the family of *Hamamelidaceae* which grows in Asia Minor and Syria. The styrax of the ancient Greeks seems to have come from *Styrax officinalis,* closely related to *Styrax benzoin,* which supplies benzoin. This styrax was a resin brought by the Phoenicians in the days of Herod to Greece and was also, therefore, the styrax of the ancient Hebrews. In the Middle Ages, styrax was understood to mean both the resin and the balsam. Both products smell of benzoin.

Myrtle Oil

When Ezra, at the behest of the people in the seventh month, brings forth the law of Moses, they read in it which kind of plants should be used to build booths:

> 'Go forth unto the mount, and fetch olive branches, and branches of wild olive, and myrtle branches, and palm branches, and branches of thick trees, to make booths, as it is written.'
> (Nehemiah 8:15)

Myrtle grew throughout Palestine and has beautiful, smooth, ovate leaves. *Myrtus communis,* from the family of *Myrtaceae,* was therefore eminently suitable for the Feast of the Tabernacles throughout Israel. The ancient Israelites used the peppery tasting berries of this plant as seasoning. Today, the essential oil is extracted from the leaves and used as a folk remedy for bladder and lung complaints.

Rose Oil

The roses referred to in the books of the Apocrypha are probably true roses from the genus *Rosa,* of the *Rosaceae.* In the passage where Jesus of Sirach proclaims the glory of wisdom, he would also have meant a true rose tree:

> There I grew like a cedar of Lebanon,
> like a cypress on the slopes of Hermon,
> like a date-palm at Engedi,
> like roses at Jericho. . . .
> (Ecclesiasticus 24:13, 14)

> Listen to me, my devout sons, and blossom
> like a rose planted by a stream.
> (Ecclesiasticus 39:13)

There were rose nurseries around Jericho and the most beautiful roses would have been found there. The rose of Media and Persia was introduced late into Palestine, only after the Babylonian captivity, approximately 560 B.C. The plant which is now known as the rose of Jericho does not belong to the genus *Rosa,* but is *Anastatica Hierochuntica,* belonging to the *Cruciferae.* This is a low desert plant with branches bent toward each other so that the whole shrub has the appearance of a ball. In autumn, the branches dry out and the trunk can be broken off by the wind, which blows this vegetable ball around.

In Bulgaria, the preparation of the fragrant oil of roses is by distillation of fresh roses in kettles of water over an open fire. This method does not appear to have been known in ancient Israel. Rose oil is particularly in demand for the preparation of perfume; it still has a place in medicine as a taste corrigent.

Spike Oil

When the bridegroom in The Song of Songs compares his bride with all kinds of lovely plants, he also mentions the nard. This plant gives the fragrant spikenard, which originally came from Arabia and India and was later also prepared in Palestine. Spikenard is now known as spike oil, which is obtained by means of distillation with vapor, from the flowers of *Lavandula spica,* a shrub from the family of *Labiatae,* native to the western Mediterranean region. *Lavandula spica* is closely related to our commonly known lavender, *Lavandula vera.* The fragrant violet-blue flowers of this shrub are placed between linen or are mixed with tobacco. The native land of the plants suggests that the "nard" of the ancient Hebrews may have been another plant. It is suspected that *Nardostachys Jatamansi,* belonging to the family of *Valerianaceae,* could have been the Biblical nard. The root and young branches of this plant, native to the West Indies and India, have a fragrant smell, and the essential oil smells a little like valerian. The nard was evidently held in high regard since the oil was falsified—an honor paid to only the most precious oils:

> Jesus was at Bethany, in the house of Simon the leper. As he sat at table, a woman came in carrying a small bottle of very costly perfume, pure oil of nard. She broke it open and poured the oil over his head.
> (Mark 14:3, 4)

Olive Oil

The olive tree, *Olea europea,* belonging to the family of *Oleaceae,* is mentioned often in the Bible. It grows wild but is also cultivated in Palestine. The western slopes of Lebanon, the coastal region and the mountain ridge of Galilee, are densely populated by these trees. The most famous grow in the garden of Gethsemane, which some say date from the time of Jesus since these trees can live to a very old age. The olive tree is mentioned at the beginning of Genesis (8:11); Noah knew that the water had subsided from the earth because of the fresh olive leaf brought back to him by the dove.

The olive competes with the grape vine and the fig tree for precedence with respect to its use to mankind; the olive tree was taken, far back in antiquity, to Greece, and from there to Italy, Southern France and later to North America. The olive tree, *sajit* in Hebrew (meaning glossy or fresh-green), is bushy when growing in the wild but can be grown to a height of 40 feet. It is evergreen and produces plumlike, black-green stone fruits: olives, the flesh of which contains 50% oil. Olive oil is collected after removing the stones and stalks of ripe olives; the fruit is then pounded to a pulp and squeezed through fine jute bags. Olive oil, which now occupies a very important place in medicine, also had a medicinal use in antiquity. It also played an important role in anointing. When kings and priests were ordained, oil was poured over their heads; even the tabernacle and all the objects were anointed with the oil that, for this purpose, was mixed with myrrh, cinnamon, calamus and cassia. (Exodus 30:22) Jacob anointed the stone which he placed under his head before going to sleep on the night when he dreamed that he saw the ladder which stretched from the earth to heaven: "... and set it up for a pillar, and poured oil upon the top of it. And he called the name of that place Beth-el..." (Genesis 28:18, 19)

It is evident from the fable told by Jotham to the men of Shechem (see Restharrow, page 18) that the olive tree, the fig tree and the grape vine were of great significance. The fact that the olive tree flourished even on bare rocks particularly made it a sought after plant. This is also indicated by:

> ... And He made him to suck honey out of the crag,
> And oil out of the flinty rock...
> (Deuteronomy 32:13)

Olive oil was also used as a source of light: "And thou shalt command the children of Israel, that they bring unto thee pure olive oil beaten for the light, to cause a lamp to burn continually." (Exodus 27:20)

Aloes

Any authority on pharmacy is always surprised that aloes, a bitter, unpleasant smelling extract from the leaves of different types of *Aloe,* should be mentioned in the same breath as myrrh and other aromatic substances: "Myrrh, and aloes, and cassia are all thy garments . . ." (Psalms 45:9)

The aloe of the Old Testament is actually a type of wood which comes from *Aloexylon,* now used for perfume in eastern countries. This wood has a very pleasant lemonlike smell and was taken from the Cochinchina mountains to Palestine for the purpose of trade. It must also have been this type of aloe which was used for burial of the dead:

> . . . so Joseph came and took the body away. He was joined by Nicodemus (the man who had first visited Jesus by night), who brought with him a mixture of myrrh and aloes, more than half a hundredweight. They took the body of Jesus and wrapped it, with the spices, in strips of linen cloth according to Jewish burial-customs.
> (John 19:39, 40)

It is quite possible that the aloe used here is the thickened sap of the leaves of types of Aloe which grew in Africa and about which the Israelites learned during their exile.

Animal Products

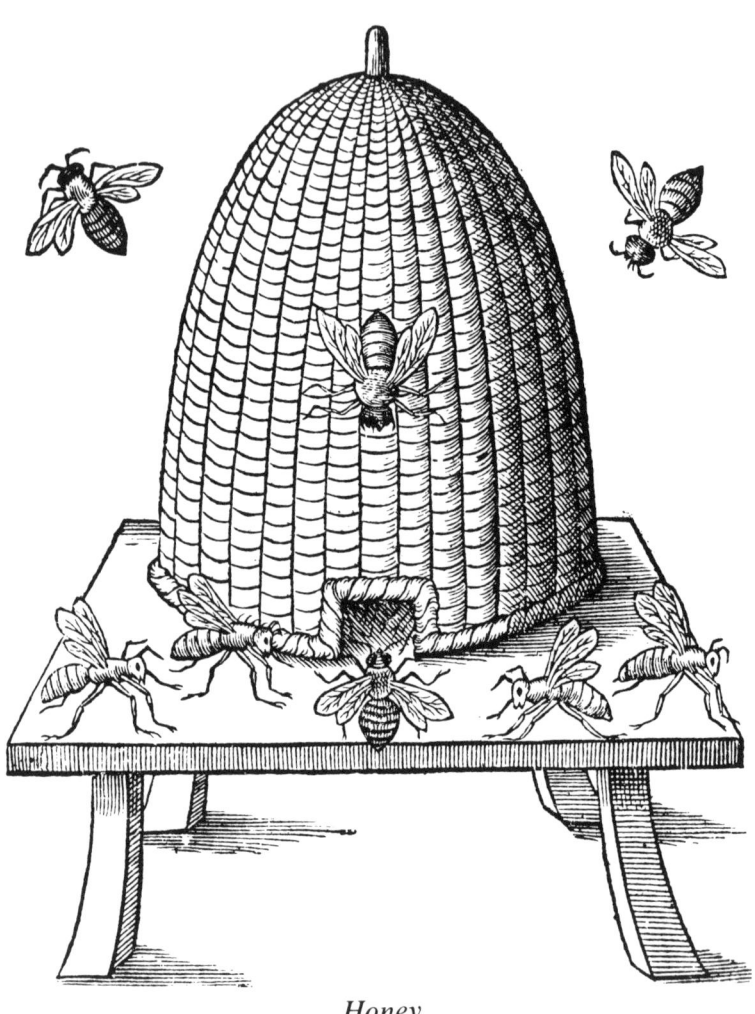

Honey

Carmine

Carmine is referred to in many passages in the Bible. It generally signifies cloth which has been dyed red with carmine. The carmine used by the ancient Hebrews comes from *Coccus Ilicis,* the kermes scale insect which lives on the kermes oak, *Quercus coccifera,* in Asia Minor. This insect is killed in boiling water or by vapor from hot water and then dried, and appears on the market as "kermes." The kermes insect contains less dye than the nopal insect, *Coccus cacti,* which originally came from Mexico and is now bred elsewhere. The dried female provides cochineal, a red dyestuff, which is used in the dyeing industry, and is also sometimes a constituent of toothpowders and ointments.

Carmine, or "scarlet," is among the offerings the Lord requests from the Israelites for building the sanctuary.

> And the Lord spoke unto Moses, saying: 'Speak unto the children of Israel, that they take for Me an offering; of every man whose heart maketh him willing ye shall take My offering. And this is the offering which ye shall take of them: gold, and silver, and brass, and blue, and purple, and scarlet, and fine linen, and goats' hair; and rams' skins dyed red, and sealskins, and acacia-wood; oil for the light, spices for the anointing oil, and for the sweet incense; onyx stones, and stones to be set, for the ephod, and for the breastplate.
> (Exodus 25:1-7)

Gall

Fish galls were used in antiquity as a medicinal remedy for eye complaints. There is no mention of which fish were used. Other animal organs were used for the treatment of illness—for example, heart and liver for insanity. Thickened oxgall, i.e. the contents of the gallbladder of an ox in the form of a thickened extract, is still used in organotherapy. The gall of a fish is used by Tobias to restore the sight of his father:

> '. . . Spread the fish-gall on his eyes, and the medicine will make the white patches shrink and peel off. Your father will get his sight back and see the light of day.'
> (Tobit 11:8)

Coral

The poet of Lamentations describes the wretched lot of the beseiged and fallen Zion, saying:

> Her princes were purer than snow,
> They were whiter than milk,
> They were more ruddy in body than rubies [or coral],
> Their polishing was as of sapphire;
> Their visage is blacker than coal;
> They are not known in the streets;
> Their skin is shrivelled upon their bones;
> It is withered, it is become like a stick.
> (Lamentations 4:7, 8)

The New English version of the Bible provides "coral" as the translation. A German Bible gives "red pearl." It is most probably coral that is indicated here since from very early times divers fished for coral on the east coast of the Mediterranean and the ancient Hebrews would certainly have known about these jewels which were obtained with such difficulty. Coral is the the chalky skeleton of the coral polyps, a low form of animal life. Red coral is occasionally used medicinally as a dye for powders.

Honey

Although honey is still a favorite food, it was of even greater importance to the ancient Hebrews since they did not know of sugar. Honey, therefore, was used for sweetening food and drink. It was used both internally and externally as a medicine and is still used as such. The term "honey" also meant the "must" from grapes, which was boiled to the thickness of syrup, and also referred to a syrup made from ripe dates. True honey comes from bees, and since no mention is made in the Bible of beehives, wild bees must have been the chief supplier. These bees made their home in hollow tree trunks and splits in the rocks; the Lord showed Israel the honey of wild bees:

> He made him ride on the high places of the earth,
> And he did eat the fruitage of the field;
> And He made him to suck honey out of the crag,
> And oil out of the flinty rock...
> (Deuteronomy 32:13)

The Bible clearly points to the presence of honey in the trees. When Jonathan, during the battle with the Philistines, eats honey despite orders from his father Saul to the contrary, it seems that the food value of honey was already known:

> So the Lord saved Israel that day; and the battle passed on as far as Beth-aven. And the men of Israel were distressed that day; but Saul adjured the people, saying: 'Cursed be the man that eateth any food until it be evening, and I be avenged on mine enemies.' So none of the people tasted food.

> And all the people came to the forest; and there was honey upon the ground. And when the people were come unto the forest, behold a flow of honey; but no man put his hand to his mouth; for the people feared the oath. But Jonathan heard not when his father charged the people with the oath; and he put forth the end of the rod that was in his hand, and dipped it in the honeycomb, and put his hand to his mouth; and his eyes brightened. Then answered one of the people, and said: 'Thy father straitly charged the people with an oath, saying: Cursed be the man that eateth food this day; and the people are faint.' Then said Jonathan: 'My father hath troubled the land; see, I pray you, how mine eyes are brightened, because I tasted a little of this honey. How much more, if haply the people had eaten, freely to-day of the spoil of their enemies which they found? had there not been then a much greater slaughter among the Philistines?'
>
> (I Samuel 14:23-30)

It is of course quite understandable that many things which were pleasant and lovely were compared with honey. In reference to the laws of the Lord, one finds:

> How sweet are Thy words unto my palate!
> Yea, sweeter than honey to my mouth!
>
> (Psalms 119:103)

Even better than honey was the honeycomb itself; it is expressed as a poignant contrast to bitterness:

> The full soul loatheth a honeycomb;
> But to the hungry soul every bitter thing is sweet.
>
> (Proverbs 27:7)

Bibliography

Buchheister-Ottersbach. Handbuch der Drogisten-praxis.
Ebstein. Die Medizin in Alten Testament.
Goester. Pharmacognosie.
Heukels. Geïllustreerde Schoolflora.
Kuenen, Hooykaas, Kosters and Oort. Het Oude Testament opnieuw uit den Grondtekst overgezet, de z.g.n. Leidsche Vertaling 1899.
Oort. Het Nieuwe Testament.
Palm, van der. Alle de Boeken des Nieuwen Verbonds 1825.
_____. De Apokryfe Boeken des Ouden Verbonds 1830.
Neuburger. Die Medizin in der Bibel. Velhagen und Klasings Monatshefte 1920.
Schelens. Geschichte der Pharmazie.
Smith. Bible Plants. 1877.
Statenvertaling van het Oude en het Nieuwe Testament.
Strasburger. Lehrbuch der Botanik.
Visser, de. Hebreeuwsche Archaeologie.
Wunderbar. Biblisch-Talmudische Medicin. 1850.
Zeller. Biblisches Wörterbuch 1866.
Zörnig. Arzneidrogen.

Index

A

Aaron, 70
Abimelech, 19
abortifacient, 43
absinthe, 49
absinthiine, 49
Acacia, 20
Acacia arabica Wildd, 31, 32
Acacia senegal, 32
acacia wood, 30, 31, 32, 84, 101
acetic acid infusion, 62
aconite root, 25
Aconitum napellus, 25
Acorus calamus, 23
alchemists, 45
alcoholic drinks, 8
alkanna root, 22
Alkanna tinctoria, 22
alkaloids, 63
Allium cepa, 26
Allium porrum, 27
Allium sativum, 25
Allium shoenoprasum L., 27
almonds, 68, 77, 78
almug tree, 33
aloes, 23, 97

Aloexylon, 97
amygdalin, 78
Amygdalus amarus, 78
Amygdalus dulcis, 78
Anacardiaceae, 88, 91
anaesthetic, 44, 86
Anastatica hierochuntica, 94
anchusa, 22
Andropogon calamus aromaticus, 24
Anethum graveolens, 69
animal gall, 62; substances, 8
antirheumatic, 48
antiseptic, 45
aphrodisiac, 52
apothecary, 9, 12
apples, 72
Araceae, 23
Ark of the Covenant, 31
aromatic, 36, 51, 89
Artemisia absinthium, 49
Asa, 5, 9
Astragalus, 20, 83
astringent, 35, 39, 66
Atropa mandragora, 17
autumn crocus corms, see crocus

B

Balanophoraceae, 21
balms, 7, 8, 9, 13, 89
balsam, 68, 85, 88, 89, 93
barley, 61, 69, 83;
 barley bread, 61, 62
baths, water, 7, 8
bdellium, 86
Benjamin, 67
benzaldehyde, 78
benzoin, 93
birch, 19
blackberry, 52
bladder, 93
blindness, 7
bloodspitting, 35
Boaz, 67
Boraginaceae, 22
Boswellia, 84
Boswellia carterii, 84, 85
bramble leaves, 52
Brassica alba, 75
Brassica nigra, 75
bronchitis, 92
broom, 60, 61;
 broom charcoal, 21;
 broom root, 20
burial rituals, 85
burns, 76
Burseraceae, 85, 86

C

calamus, 24, 96;
 calamus root, 23;
 calamus, sweet, 9
Canaan, 64
cancer, treatment of, 45
Cannabinaceae, 44
Cannabis sativa, 44
caper buds, 54
Capparidaceae, 54
Capparis spinosa, 20, 48, 54
Carduus marianus, 77
caries, 7
carmine, 101
cassia, 9, 23, 36, 53, 96, 97
castor-oil plant, 76, 77
caterpillars, 77
cathartic, 77
cedar, 32, 47, 92
cedrus libani, 91
celandine, 45
chelidon, 45
chelidonium, 45
chives, 27
Cinnamomum cassia, 35
cinnamon, 9, 23, 35, 36, 96
circumcision, 69
Cistaceae, 90
Cistus creticus, 90
Citrius medica L., 63
Citrullus colocynthis, 72
Citrus Limonum Risso, 63
cleansing rites, 47
cloth, 37
cloves, 53, 54
Coccus cacti, 101
Coccus ilicis, 101
codeine, 62
colchicum autumnale, 24
colic, 35
colocynth apples, 72, 73
colophonium, 87, 88
Commiphora abyssinica, 85
Commiphora africana, 86

common wormwood, 49
Compositae, 77
compresses, for bleeding, 66
confinements, 6
Coniferae, 43, 60, 87, 91
coniine, 46
Conium maculatum, 46
Convallaria majalis, 25
coral, 102, 103
coriander, 68, 82
Coriandrum sativum, 68
corn plaster, 44
cotton, 37, 38, 81
crocus corms, 24
Crocus sativus, 52, 53
crown of thorns, 20
Cruciferae, 75, 94
cucumbers, 25, 74; wild, 73
Cucumis citrullus, 74
Cucumis melo, 74
Cucumis sativus, 74
Cucurbitaceae, 73, 74
Cupuliferae, 35
cummin, 68, 69
Cuminum cyminum, 68
currant, 64, 65
Cynomorium coccineum, 21
cypress, 32

D

dates, 8, 36, 59
date palm, 60
David, 87, 88
deadly nightshade, 17
delirium, 49
diarrhea, 52
dietary remedy, 27
dill, 69
disinfectant, 92
diuretic, 52
druggists, 12
dye, 103
dysentery, 7

E

Elijah, 4, 21
Elisha, 4, 8, 73
Ericaceae, 43
essential oil, 23, 43, 49, 51, 54, 64, 69, 75, 86, 91, 92, 93, 95
Eugenia caryophyllata, 54
expectorant, 48
external remedy, 71
extract, herbal, 10
eye complaints, 45, 102; eye remedy, 8, 11
Ezra, 93

F

fertility, 38
Ferula galbaniflua, 87
fever, 7
Ficus carica, 71
figs, 65, 70, 71, 96
fir tree, 87
fishgall, 8, 62, 102
flax, 76
foetentes, 26
fragrant oils, 9
frankincense, 9, 24, 84, 85
Fraxinus ornus, 82
freckles, 45

fresh water, 8
fungus melitensis, 21

G

galban, 53
galbanum, 9, 86, 87
gall, 86, 102
gallbladder, 102
gallfly, 35, 81
gallnuts, 35, 81
garlic, 25, 26, 74
gastric remedy, 52
Genista raetem, 20, 21
Genista scoparia Lamk, 21
gin, 61
glucoside, 34, 75, 78
glue, 89
Gossypium, 81;
   gossypium bark, 27
Gossypium herbaceum, 37
Gossypium hirsutum, 37
Gossypium religiosum, 37
gout, 51
Graminaceae, 61
Graminae, 83
grapes, 8; grapevine, 64, 96
greater celandine, 45, 77
gum arabic, 32
gum resin, 53, 84, 86
gum tragacanth, 68, 83

H

hallucinogen, 49
Hamamelidaceae, 93

health practices, 3, 4, 8
heart remedy, 26
heather, 21, 43
hemlock, 46
hemp, 44
henna flowers, 22
herbal mixtures, 9, 11
Hezekiah, King, 11, 71
holy anointing oil, 9, 10, 24,
   35, 36, 38, 96, 101
holy water sprinkler, 47
homeopathy, 45
honey, 8, 11, 68, 82, 89, 103,
   104
Hordeum distichum, 61
Hordeum vulgare, 61
Hosea, 46
husked barley, 61
hygiene, 3, 7, 8
hypochondria, 26
hyssop, 47, 48, 91
Hyssopus officinalis, 48

I

illness, 3, 7, 27
incense, 9, 31, 38, 53, 84, 101
indian hemp, 44
inflammation, 71; of urinary
   organs, 76
internal remedy, 71
intestinal remedy, 52, 89
Iridaceae, 52
Iris florentina, 23
iris root, 23, 36
Isaiah, 4, 18, 71

J

Jacob, 4, 50, 67, 78, 83, 96
jaundice, 45, 77
Jeremiah, 7, 24, 43, 78
Jesus, 6, 12, 46, 51, 86, 95
Jezebel, 21
Job, 21, 44
Joseph, 4, 17, 67, 83, 89
Joshua, 76
Jotham, 19, 96
Juglandaceae, 51
Juglans regia, 51
juniper, 43, 60, 61
Juniperus communis, 43, 60
Juniperus sabina, 43
Juniperus virginiana, 91

K

kermes, 101
kermes scale insect, 101
kidney stones, 18

L

Laban, 50
labdanum, 89, 90
labiate, 48
Labiatae, 48, 51, 95
ladanum, 13, 89
larch tree, 32
Lauraceae, 36, 51
laurel leaves, 51
Laurus nobilis, 51

lavender, 95
Lavandula spica, 95
Lavandula vera, 95
law of Moses, 3, 4, 5, 93
Lawsonia inermis, 22
laxative, 26, 71
Leah, 17
leek, 26
Leguminosae, 33
lemon peel, 63, 64
leper, ritual cleansing of, 47, 91, 92
leprosy, 7
Levites, 4
Liliaceae, 25, 26, 27
lily of the valley, 25
Linaceae, 76
linen, 37, 38, 76
linseed, 76; linseed meal, 71
Linum usitasissimum, 76
Liguidambar orientalis, 92
love potions, 17
lubricant, 77
lung complaints, 93
Lythraceae, 22

M

Malvaceae, 37
mandrake root, 17
manna, 26, 68, 81, 82
mannatol, 82
marjoram, 48
mastic, 88, 89, 91
medicine, 7ff, 12
melancholy, 26
melons, 25

mental disorders, 7
Mentha, 51
Mentha piperita, 52
menthol, 51
methods of healing, 7
midwives, 6
migraine, 51
milk, to stimulate production, 45
milk thistle seed, 77
Mimosaceae, 31
mint, 51, 69
miraculous cures, 4
monkshood, 25
Moraceae, 70, 71
morphine, 62
Morus alba, 70
Morus nigra, 70
Moses, 35, 36, 47, 53, 70
mulberries, 70
mustard paper, 75; plaster, 75; seed, 75
myrrh, 9, 23, 53, 68, 83, 84, 85, 86, 89, 96, 97
Myrtaceae, 54, 93
myrtle, 32, 59; oil, 93
Myrtus communis, 93

N

narcissus, 25
narcotic remedy, 44, 62
nard, 95
Nardostachys Jatamansi, 95
Noah, 64, 95
nurse, 6

O

oak apples, 35, 81
oak bark, 34, 35, 81
oil, 8, 9, 10, 11, 12, 23, 32, 37, 38, 63, 89
ointments, 11, 32, 101
Oleaceae, 82, 95
Olea europea, 95
oleum cinnamomi, 36
oleum santali, 33
olibanum, 84
olive, 59, 93, 96; oil, 9, 95
onion, 26
Ononis antiquorem, 18
Ononis spinosa, 18
onycha, 9
onyx, 53, 86, 101
opium, 62, 63
Origanum aegypticum, 48
oxgall, 62, 102

P

pain-killing drugs, 8, 47, 62, 75
paint, 88
palm, 59, 60, 63, 93
Palmae, 59
Papaveraceae, 62
Papaver setigerum DC, 62
Papaver somniferum L., 62
Papilionaceae, 18, 21, 83
paralysis, 7
pears, 72
Pentateuch, 3
peppermint leaves, 51, 69

perfume, 9, 10, 22, 23, 32, 53, 85, 86, 89, 90, 92, 94, 95, 97
Phoenix dactylifera, 59
physician, 4, 5, 6, 12
pine tree, 87, 88
Pinus, 87, 91
Pinus silvestris, 88
Pistacia Lentiscus, 88, 91
Pistacia terebinthus, 67, 91
Pistacia vera, 67, 91
pistachio nuts, 67, 68
plague, 7
plasters, 87, 88
poisonous plants, 24, 25, 46, 78
pomegranate, 50, 64, 71; bark, 38
poplar buds, 50
poppy capsules, 62
populus, 50
Populus nigra, 50
poultice, 76
Prunus amygdalus, 78
prussic acid, 78
Pterocarpus santalinus, 33
Punicaceae, 39
Punica granatum, 39
purgative, 8, 73
Pyrus malus, 72

Q

Quercus coccifera, 101
Quercus infectoria, 35
Quercus sessiflora, 35
quinces, 72

R

Rachel, 17
Rahab, 76
raisin, 64, 65
Ranunculaceae, 25
red dye, 22
resin, 12, 44, 85, 86, 87, 88, 89, 91, 93
Reuben, 17
Rhamnaceae, 20
rheumatism, 75, 89
rheumatic lumbago, 66
Ricinus communis, 76
ricinus seed, 76, 77
Rosa, 93, 94
Rosaceae, 52, 72, 78, 93
rose, 25, 94; oil, 93, 94
Rubus fructuosus, 52
rue, 45, 46, 51
Rutaceae, 45, 63
Ruta graveolene, 45
Ruth, 67

S

sabine, 43
saffron, 52, 53
Salicaceae, 34
salicin, 34
saliylic acid, 34
Salix alba, 33
Salix fragilis, 33
sandalwood, 32, 33; oil, 91
Santalum album, 33
Santalaceae, 33
santonin, 49

scabies, 7
scurvy grass, 86
Serothamnus scoparius, 21
sessile oak, 35
silkworms, 70
Sirach, 4, 5, 12, 13, 53
sirupus mororum, 70
skin diseases, 7, 22, 83
smoking, 8
Solanaceae, 17
Solomon, 92
Spartium scoparium L., 21
spearmint, 51
spices, 9, 12, 13, 33, 38
spikenard, 94
spike oil, 94, 95
spiny restharrow root, 18
sprinkles, 47
stacte, 9, 92
starch, 61
stimulant, 54, 60
stinging nettle, 44
St. Luke, 6
St. Matthew, 48
stomachic, 54, 61, 69
styptic, 35
styrax, 90, 92, 93
Styrax benzoin, 93
Styrax officinalis, 92, 93
sweet root, 35

T

Tamaricaceae, 82
tamarisk, 81, 82
Tamarix mannifera, 82
Tamr-el-Hinna, 22

tannic acid, 35
tanning, 34, 39
taste corrigent, 68, 70, 94
teeth, 67
terebinth, 34, 35, 90
Theophrastus, 63, 76
thistle, 77
thornbush, 18, 19, 20
thorn in the eye, 20
thorns, 18, 19
tinctures, 11
toothache, 66, 86
toothpowder, 32, 101
tragacanth, 83
Triticum vulgare, 83
tuberculosis, 7
tumors, 63
turpentine, 67, 88, 90, 91

U

ulceration, 71
ulcers, 83, 90
Umbelliferae, 68, 69, 87
Urticaceae, 45
Urtica dioica, 45
Urtica urens, 45

V

valerian, 95
Valerianaceae, 95
varnish, 32, 88, 89
vegetable oils, 8
veneral disease, 89

vermicidal, 26, 39, 49
vinegar, 11, 48, 54, 66, 67
Vitaceae, 65
vitis vinifera, 65
volatile oil, 24, 26, 45, 49, 85

wine, 8, 19, 54, 59, 60, 64, 65, 66, 86
worm diseases, 7, 26, 51
wormwood, 49

W

walnut leaves, 50 51
warts, 45
washings, 8
water baths, 7, 8
wax, 12
wheat, 69, 83, 89
willow, 63; bark, 33, 50

Y

yellow dye, 22

Z

Zizyphus, 20
Zizyphus spina Christi, 20